Abnormalities in Puberty

Scientific and Clinical Advances

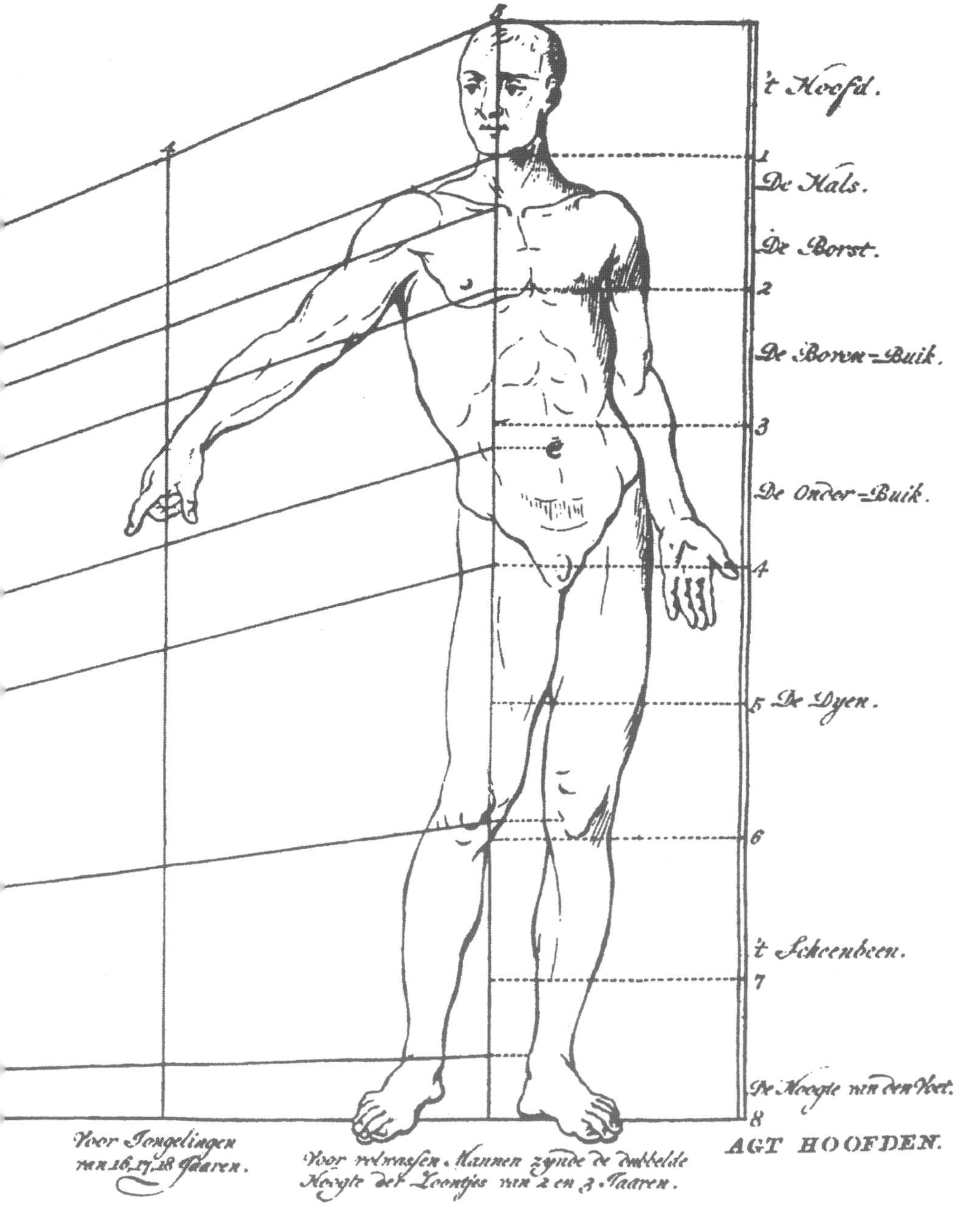

Endocrine Development

Vol. 8

Series Editor

Martin O. Savage *London*

KARGER

Abnormalities in Puberty

Scientific and Clinical Advances

Volume Editor

Henriette A. Delemarre-van de Waal *Amsterdam*

41 figures, 2 in color, and 11 tables, 2005

KARGER

Basel · Freiburg · Paris · London · New York ·
Bangalore · Bangkok · Singapore · Tokyo · Sydney

Prof. Dr. Henriette A. Delemarre-van de Waal
VU University Medical Center
Paediatric Endocrinology
PO Box 7057
Amsterdam, The Netherlands

Library of Congress Cataloging-in-Publication Data

Abnormalities in puberty : scientific and clinical advances / volume editor,
Henriette A. Delemarre-van de Waal.
p. ; cm. – (Endocrine development, ISSN 1421-7082 ; v. 8)
Includes bibliographical references and indexes.
ISBN 3-8055-7867-9 (hard cover : alk. paper)
1. Pediatric endocrinology. 2. Endocrine glands–Diseases. 3. Precocious puberty. 4. Puberty.
[DNLM: 1. Puberty, Precocious. 2. Gonadal Disorders. 3. Puberty, Delayed. 4. Puberty. WS 450 A153 2005] I. Delemarre-van de Waal, H. A. (Henriette A.) II. Series.
RJ418.A24 2005
618.92′4–dc22

2004026715

Bibliographic Indices. This publication is listed in bibliographic services, including Current Contents® and Index Medicus.

Drug Dosage. The authors and the publisher have exerted every effort to ensure that drug selection and dosage set forth in this text are in accord with current recommendations and practice at the time of publication. However, in view of ongoing research, changes in government regulations, and the constant flow of information relating to drug therapy and drug reactions, the reader is urged to check the package insert for each drug for any change in indications and dosage and for added warnings and precautions. This is particularly important when the recommended agent is a new and/or infrequently employed drug.

www.karger.com
Printed in Switzerland on acid-free paper by Reinhardt Druck, Basel
ISSN 1421–7082
ISBN 3–8055–7867–9

Contents

VII Foreword
Savage, M.O. (London)

IX Preface
Delemarre-van de Waal, H.A. (Amsterdam)

1 Secular Trend of Timing of Puberty
Delemarre-van de Waal, H.A. (Amsterdam)

15 Fetal Nutrition and Timing of Puberty
van Weissenbruch, M.M.; Engelbregt, M.J.T.; Veening, M.A.; Delemarre-van de Waal, H.A. (Amsterdam)

34 Adrenal Function of Low-Birthweight Children
Ong, K. (Cambridge)

54 Puberty and Fertility in Congenital Adrenal Hyperplasia
Otten, B.J.; Stikkelbroeck, M.M.L.; Claahsen-van der Grinten, H.L.; Hermus, A.R.M.M. (Nijmegen)

67 Molecular Genetics of Isolated Hypogonadotropic Hypogonadism and Kallmann Syndrome
Karges, B. (Ulm); de Roux, N. (Paris)

81 Hypothalamic Hamartoma: A Paradigm/Model for Studying the Onset of Puberty
Jung, H.; Parent, A.-S.; Ojeda, S.R. (Beaverton, Oreg.)

94 **Gonadotropin-Releasing Hormone Analogue Treatment for Precocious Puberty.** Twenty Years of Experience
Heger, S.; Sippell, W.G. (Kiel); Partsch, C.-J. (Esslingen)

126 **Very Long-Term Follow-Up of Girls with Early and Late Menarche**
Johansson, T.; Ritzén, E.M. (Örebro)

137 **Polycystic Ovary Syndrome in Adolescence.**
New Insights in Pathophysiology and Treatment
Homburg, R. (Amsterdam)

150 **Reversing Sex Steroid Deficiency and Optimizing Skeletal Development in the Adolescent with Gonadal Failure**
Vanderschueren, D.; Vandenput, L.; Boonen, S. (Leuven)

166 **Present and Future Options for the Preservation of Fertility in Female Adolescents with Cancer**
Beerendonk, C.C.M.; Braat, D.D.M. (Nijmegen)

176 **Author Index**

177 **Subject Index**

Foreword

I am delighted to announce the publication of another important issue in the *Endocrine Development* series. This volume presents new clinical and scientific data on a subject of major clinical and physiological interest, namely abnormalities of puberty. Professor Henriette A. Delemarre-van de Waal, who has acknowledged expertise both as a clinician and basic scientist, has skillfully assembled an impressive group of contributors. The volume includes topics of great interest, including several that are infrequently discussed such as fetal nutrition and timing of puberty, adrenal function in low-birth-weight children and puberty in congenital adrenal hyperplasia.

Other subjects of direct clinical relevance are covered, such as experience with GnRH analogue therapy, polycystic ovary syndrome, consequences of early and late puberty, growth associated with gonadal failure and preservation of fertility in the cancer patient. The volume is completed with several erudite yet clearly explained chapters on the molecular genetics of Kallmann's syndrome and the physiology of the onset of puberty.

This is a very well balanced edition. The contents are clearly set out and easily readable. I am confident that this worthy addition to the series will prove of great value to pediatric and adult endocrinologists and to all health workers concerned with puberty, the crucial phase of development and transition from childhood to adult life.

M.O. Savage

Preface

Over recent decades new insights have been obtained surrounding the concepts of the regulation of the onset of puberty. However, human puberty remains a mystery. The mechanisms responsible for suppression and reawakening of the GnRH pulse generator from fetal life into puberty still need to be elucidated. However, many genetic and environmental factors have been identified modulating the pubertal process.

This book on the abnormalities of puberty gives an overview on the latest knowledge in the physiology and pathophysiology of puberty and its disorders. Are there consequences for clinical practice on the findings of a continued trend of an earlier puberty in the United States? What are the underlying mechanisms of an early puberty in adopted children? We know that early growth, during the fetal period as well as during childhood, is able to program the central regulatory system related to growth, adrenarche and puberty. Endocrine and metabolic issues related to the 'developmental origin of adult disease' hypothesis and to the polycystic ovary syndrome are discussed. Abnormalities in GnRH release controlling genes are reviewed. The hamartoma, secreting GnRH, is described as a model of the onset of puberty. Experience on the application of GnRH analogues in the treatment of central precocious puberty as well as the psychosocial effects of an early puberty are extensively reported.

How should one treat the patient with gonadal failure with respect to bone development in order to prevent osteoporosis in later life and what are the future perspectives with respect to preservation of fertility in later life?

Recent clinical and fundamental data are described to give you an update on the new views on the control of puberty. We intend to support clinicians in the management of the child with too early onset of puberty, with delayed puberty and other pubertal disorders. Not only the clinical aspects, but also the aspects related to their causes such as early growth, and genetic and developmental defects are discussed, which may have consequences on final height, bone development and reproduction.

Henriette A. Delemarre-van de Waal

Delemarre-van de Waal HA (ed): Abnormalities in Puberty. Scientific and Clinical Advances.
Endocr Dev. Basel, Karger, 2005, vol 8, pp 1–14

Secular Trend of Timing of Puberty

Henriette A. Delemarre-van de Waal

VU University Medical Center, Amsterdam, The Netherlands

Abstract

During the last decades, a secular trend of growth and timing of puberty occurred consisting of increased adult height and earlier onset of puberty. In The Netherlands although the most recent survey showed an increase of final height again, the timing of puberty onset appears to level off, and in boys pubertal onset was even slightly retarded.

Different findings were reported from the United States, where a strong advancement of the onset of puberty was observed in both white and black girls, although the effect was more evident in black girls.

Timing of puberty follows a familial pattern and therefore seems to be controlled by genetic factors, whereas environmental factors may influence and mediate the genetic regulation. Environmental factors such as nutritional status, chronic diseases, migration to a healthy environment, frequent infectious diseases, pollution and exposure to insecticides are all thought to influence the endocrine regulation status and therefore differentiation and development of endocrine organs. In this chapter, the physiologic mechanisms of puberty onset with the different regulatory aspects, as well as pathologic processes interfering with the onset of puberty will be discussed.

Puberty is the result of increasing gonadotropin-releasing hormone (GnRH) release by the hypothalamus followed by a complex sequence of endocrine changes with functioning of negative and positive feedback, and is associated with the development of sex characteristics, a growth spurt and reproductive competence. During the fetal period the GnRH-gonadotropin axis is already functioning as can be observed by the high levels of both luteinizing hormone (LH) and follicle-stimulating hormone (FSH) at mid-gestation when the development of the vascular portal system has completed. This mid-gestational peak is followed by a decline of gonadotropin levels presumably the result of a developing negative feedback as well as due to central inhibiting influences on GnRH release [1].

Gonadotropin levels are low at birth, which is followed by a transient increase during the first months of life, the so-called postnatal peak. Thereafter, levels return into a very low, often undetectable range during the prepubertal phase as a result of the instrinsic restraint. This developmental pattern of the gonadotropin axis appears to be independent of the fetal and child's own gonadal steroids, since a similar development can be observed in agonadal patients [2].

During the fetal period a sex dimorphism in gonadotropin concentrations is manifest at both the pituitary and peripheral level with higher levels in the female fetus [3]. The sex dimorphism maintains in later life. The high incidence of idiopathic central precocious puberty in girls, and the easier response of the pituitary to stimulation with GnRH in girls compared to boys are good examples of this phenomenon [4]. It is assumed that the restraint of GnRH and gonadotropin release is more intense in boys than in girls. The fact that GnRH is not completely suppressed in girls has been confirmed in a study measuring estrogens using ultra-sensitive assays to measure estrogens, showing measurable and bioactive estrogen levels in the prepubertal girl [5].

Timing of Puberty

The clinical signs of puberty are an increase of testicular volume above 3 ml (G2) in boys, and bud-shaped elevation of the areola and papilla (B2) in girls. In girls, this stage is associated with an immediate increase of height velocity, whereas in boys the pubertal spurt occurs in the second half of puberty. Girls experience menarche, a milestone of pubertal development, about 2.3 years after start of breast growth. The appearance of axillary and pubic hair is not a good measure of puberty since it depends on adrenal steroids in girls and at least initially in boys.

Improvement of the socioeconomic status appears to advance and shorten pubertal development. In the Netherlands, in the 16th to 18th centuries menarche was reported to occur at 14–15 years of age and seldom before the age of 13 years [6]. In 1928, a shift to a menarcheal age of 13.7 years was described, and in 1965 it was 13.4 years of age. The growth survey of 1980 showed that most stages of sexual maturation were reached at a younger age and menarche was again advanced to 13.3 years and in 1997 to 13.2 years.

In several European countries the trend to an earlier start of pubertal maturation seems to have come to a halt during the last decades. In the Netherlands pubertal onset even tended to be slightly later. In girls the start of breast development started at mean ages of 10.5 and 10.7 in 1980 and in 1997, respectively, whereas in boys testicular development started at the ages of 11.3 and 11.4 years in the same studies [7].

In contrast to the Dutch data, investigations in the United States have shown an ongoing trend of earlier onset of breast development in girls and genital growth in boys, particularly in the black population [8, 9]. These reports resulted in wide discussions, firstly on the methods used in these studies and secondly on whether we should adjust our criteria for the definitions of an abnormal puberty, especially for central precocious puberty.

These studies described breast development at the age of 7 years in 5% of white American girls and as high as in 15% in African-American girls. Menarche at a mean age of 12.7 years did not advance, indicating that with an earlier start but a similar menarcheal age, pubertal development in American girls progresses at a slower pace. The earlier onset of puberty in these girls is associated with an increased body mass index, which is more pronounced in white than in black girls [10]. The reason that overweight children often have an early onset of puberty may be explained by the fact that estrogens are stored in body fat resulting in increased bioactivity.

Mechanisms

The underlying mechanism of the timing of puberty is the result of a genetic constitution and the influence of environmental forces on it. Chronic malnutrition will not allow the body to spend energy in growth and puberty and fertility. The different aspects of genetic background as well as of various environmental such as malnutrition, immigration and the effects of endocrine disrupters will be discussed.

Genetics

It is well known that timing of puberty has a familial inheritance. The identification of genetic factors involved is still insufficient. Over the last decades, gene mutations playing a role in the puberty cascade are identified explaining abnormal pubertal development.

Mutations in gonadotropin genes and gonadotropin receptors have been found [for review, see 11, 12]. LH and FSH, together with TSH and hCG, are part of the family of glycoprotein hormones consisting of a common α-subunit and a hormone specific β-subunit. The α-subunit consists of 92 amino acids and is encoded by one gene localized on chromosome 6q12.21. For the

FSH β-subunit the gene is localized on 11p13. The gene encoding for the LH β-subunit is located on chromosome 19q13.32, where hCG β-subunit genes are identified as well.

Glycoproteins bind to receptors with similar structures. These receptors belong to the G protein-coupled receptors with a, for them, characteristic large extracellular hormone-binding domain at the N-terminus. The LH receptor is encoded by a gene located at chromosome 2p21. The FSH receptor gene is located on the same chromosome 2p21–16. It is evident that mutations in the gonadotropin genes and their receptors can lead to a disturbed pubertal maturation.

A mutation of the LHβ gene has been reported in a 17-year-old boy with delayed puberty. The history of his family revealed several male relatives with infertility. The boy had low testosterone levels and increased serum LH levels, which lack LH bioactivity [13]. Substitution with hCG resulted in appropriate testosterone levels, testicular growth and spermatogenesis. The boy was homozygous for this mutation, while his mother, sister and three uncles appeared to be heterozygous. The heterozygous individuals had less bioactive LH activity related to its immunoreactivity as well.

Polymorphisms as a genetic variation of the LHβ gene are also described. One of these polymorphisms leads to diminished levels of immunoreactive LH, while a bioassay measures appropriate activity. The frequency of the variant-LHβ gene appears to be high worldwide with a high frequency in Northern European countries (allelic frequency 10%) and a low frequency in Asian populations and American Indians (2.5–5%) [14]. A wide variety of phenotypes has been described, in women varying from no symptoms to recurrent miscarriages, menstrual irregularity and polycystic ovary syndrome, and in boys low testosterone levels associated with high LH levels with delayed pubertal maturation [15]. Another LHβ gene polymorphism, whereby glycine has been replaced by serine at amino acid 102, appears to be associated with an increased risk to infertility in both males and females [16, 17].

For the FSHβ gene different inactivating mutations have been described in males and females. In males, azoospermia with and without pubertal delay has been described. These men have low FSH, increased LH and low testosterone levels. DNA sequencing showed among others a homozygous 2-bp deletion in codon 61 [18]. In females, a similar as well as a different homozygous genetic condition are reported associated with an absence of FSH, low estradiol levels, lack of development of secondary sex characteristics and primary amenorrhea [19].

For both LH and FSH receptors activating and inactivating mutations of the encoding genes have been identified. A well-known activating mutation of the LH receptor is seen in the clinical syndrome of testotoxicosis, a gonadotropin-independent state of male precocious puberty characterized by slight testicular growth, virilization with increased testosterone levels and low gonadotropin levels. This condition is male limited and has an autosomal-dominant pattern of inheritance [20]. In addition to polymorphisms of the LH receptor, different kinds of inactivating mutations of the type of insertion, missense, deletion and nonsense, while for activating mutations only missense types have been described [for review, see 11].

The clinical picture of inactivating mutations of the LH receptor is different in males and females. It usually presents with a relatively mild phenotype in females with normal development of pubertal characteristics and amenorrhea, with increased LH and FSH, and low estradiol levels and no response to hCG. In contrast, males have incomplete male differentiation of external genitalia due to low testosterone levels during pregnancy. The hCG test shows a blunted testosterone response. The severity of ambiguity depends on the amount of LH receptor activity and may vary from micropenis to severe hypospadia to a complete female phenotype [21].

In contrast to the LH receptor, only a few FSH receptor mutations have been described. All polymorphisms, inactivating mutations and the only activating FSH mutation described are of the missense type. The female phenotype of homozygous FSH receptor mutation genotype consists of gonadal dysgenesis with lack of development of sex characteristics, high levels of LH and FSH, although the ovaries contain follicles [22]. In men, the phenotype is characterized by impaired testicular growth, normal virilization and often oligospermia. The gonadotropin levels are in the normal or elevated range [23].

The only activating FSH receptor mutation has been described in a man with multiple pituitary hormone deficiencies including gonadotropins. Under testosterone treatment, he developed spermatogenesis. Screening of the FSH receptor gene revealed a mutation in the transmembrane domain-encoding exon 10 [24].

At the hypothalamic level, GnRH release can be affected by genetic disorders as well. The KAL1 gene located in the Xp22.3 region encodes for a protein anosmin that shares homology with molecules involved in neuronal migration and axonal path finding. Mutations of the KAL1 gene will result in an arrest of migration of both the olfactory and GnRH neurons leading to the clinical picture of hypogonadotropic hypogonadism associated with anosmia, the Kallmann syndrome [25]. Recently, autosomal inheritance has been described among others to be due to a mutation of the fibroblastic growth factor receptor gene [26].

Congenital adrenal hypoplasia can be associated with hypogonadotropic hypogonadism and caused by DAX-1 mutations at Xp21. The congenital adrenal hypoplasia presents already during infancy, while lack of pubertal onset will become clear at a pubertal age. In some of the boys puberty can be induced by pulsatile GnRH administration, whereas others show hardly any response. The heterogeneity of responses to GnRH stimulation does suggest that both hypothalamic and pituitary defects are involved in DAX-1 mutations.

Recently, the GPR54 gene has been described as a regulator of control of puberty [27]. The GPR54 gene is a G protein-coupled receptor gene, which causes idiopathic hypogonadotropic hypogonadism in humans and mice. GPR54-deficient male mice have small testes and the female mice have a delayed vaginal opening with impaired follicular maturation. Both males and females respond adequately to exogenous gonadotropins. Hypothalamic extracts of these GPR54-deficient mice showed similar GnRH concentrations as observed in nonmutants. At the pituitary levels LH and FSH was present, indicating that the gonadotropic cells are developed, which was confirmed by responses to exogenous GnRH. These data provide strong evidence that the GPR54 gene is a key regulator in the control of puberty. However, the exact mechanisms are still unknown. Based on the described observations, the gene may play a role in either the regulation of GnRH release at the hypothalamic level or it is involved in the pituitary response to released GnRH.

Loss of function of the GnRH receptor will also result in impaired pubertal development. A variety of phenotypes has been described in affected subjects. Inactivating GnRH receptor mutations are described, which are transmitted in a recessive trait. In familial cases of hypogonadotropic hypogonadism, 50% show a loss of the GnRH receptor function [28].

In conclusion, various genetic abnormalities are described resulting in abnormalities of the hypothalamic-gonadal axis. However, whether these genes play a role in the physiologic variations in timing of puberty remains uncertain.

Nutrition

In 1971, Frisch and Revelle [29] proposed the critical weight hypothesis saying that a minimal weight is needed to achieve menarche. In their study, they observed that a mean weight of 48 kg at menarche did not alter when menarcheal age decreased, whereas mean height significantly increased. Later on, both animal and human studies indicate that a particular ratio of fat to lean body mass is necessary for the start of puberty and for maintenance of reproductive capacity. In 1973, Ruf [30] wondered 'how the brain can be informed of the nutritional state of the organism and how it "knows" when to initiate the process of puberty'. Today, we know that leptin is one of the factors informing the brain about the peripheral energy stores. Leptin is produced and secreted by white adipose tissue and has potent effects on feeding behavior, thermogenesis and neuroendocrine processes. In the case of leptin deficiency, as in the ob/ob mice, obesity and infertility occur. Replacement of leptin will decrease the food intake and restore reproductive function. Leptin exerts its effects via the NPY neurons. It decreases NPY signalling by acting directly on the NPY-containing perikarya and presumably also at the level of the NPY nerve terminals.

In the fasting state, leptin levels decline and gonadotropin release is suppressed. Such findings suggest that nutrition contributes to pubertal development. However, it remains uncertain whether leptin is essential for the triggering of pubertal onset. Data in the rat have shown that leptin levels remain constant during the pre- and postpubertal stages. In addition, leptin gene expression in the hypothalamus does not show any developmental changes. These data suggest that leptin itself is not a strong metabolic trigger for the onset of puberty, but that it acts as a permissive signal for the onset of puberty [31].

The question arises whether the earlier onset of puberty in obese children is the result of an increased bioactivity by estrogens stored in fat, or the result of neuroendocrine modulation via leptin and NPY activities [10].

States of chronic disease associated with a low body weight are frequently accompanied by delayed puberty. A similar picture is seen in patients with anorexia nervosa; in general a depressive condition is associated with delayed puberty and failure to grow. Improvement of these physical and psychological problems, especially with respect to weight, allows normalization of the different endocrine axes including pubertal maturation.

Intrauterine Growth

Impaired fetal growth is associated with an increased risk of developing short stature, type 2 diabetes, hypertension and cardiovascular disease as a result of a changed programming in the differentiation and functioning of different organs [32]. With respect to puberty, earlier onset, more rapid progression, and increased prevalence of polycystic ovary disease and premature adrenarche have been described [33, 34]. A sexual dimorphism in the relation of birth weight and timing of puberty is reported as well, with an early onset in girls and a delayed onset in boys with decreasing birth weight [35]. Gonadal dysfunction is observed in both human and rat models. Ovarian function is impaired in adolescent girls with a low birth weight, whereas in males subfertility is more frequent [36, 37].

Perinatal malnutrition in rats leading to intrauterine growth failure is associated with delayed puberty and with a lower number of developing follicles. Postnatal food restriction has no effect on the timing of puberty, but does affect ovarian development as is seen in the increased number of growing follicles without ovulation [38, 39].

There is growing evidence that both fetal and postnatal growth exert an effect on developing organs and therefore ontogeny of diseases in later life. With respect to the fetal origin hypothesis of adult disease Ong et al. [40, 41] show that in addition to birth weight, a rapid increase of weight during infancy is strongly related to insulin resistance as well as to adrenal androgen secretion in both girls and boys.

Immigration

In children adopted from developing countries, onset of puberty often occurs at an earlier age than in their countries of origin. Prepubertal growth is often better then expected, but early puberty compromises final height [42]. However, it is good to realize that adult height in these adopted individuals is not different from those adults in the countries the children originate from [43]. As a rule, short stature is associated with a delay of puberty. Adopted children, however, have short stature at the time of adoption, but show catch up during the first years of life in their new country. The question arises whether the phenomenon of an early puberty may be a 'correction' on transient overgrowth in an individual with a different growth pattern programmed in early life. In fact, this condition is the opposite of delayed puberty, which occurs in the case of chronic disease, whereby the genetic growth potential will be maintained by a late puberty. The only way for adopted children to achieve the originally 'programmed' adult height is an earlier onset of puberty. A secular trend with increased height due to improved living circumstances is not observed in the same generation, but probably this phenomenon needs more time.

Endocrine Disrupters

Increasing exposure to endocrine disrupters, environmental substances with sex steroid agonistic and antagonistic effects, result in harmful interference from sex differentiation to male and female reproduction [44]. DDT-derived pesticides are still used in developing countries. Increased levels of DDT have been found in adopted girls with early puberty [45]. The mechanisms involved in DDT disruptions are not clear. Due to its sex steroid activity, DDT exposure may result in premature hypothalamic maturation. Another theory is that estrogen activity may suppress hypothalamic activity, while after migration, when exposure to DDT has discontinued, a drop in suppression may elicit a countereffect and therefore increased GnRH release.

Adverse environmental influences also affect male development. During the last decennia, the incidence of hypospadia and undescended testes appears to increase. In adult men this may have led to decreased semen quality and fertility [46]. The bioactivity of these drugs appears to maintain for a long period of time. This can be explained by storage of these drugs in fat and other tissues or by a persistent effect by a changed programming of different organs. Generation studies should give more insight as to how environmental influences interfere with development and reproduction.

Puberty Disorders

In Europe, precocious puberty is defined in girls as a start of breast development below the age of 8 years, and in boys growth of testes with a volume equal to or more than 4ml below the age of 9 years [47]. The studies of Herman-Giddens and coworkers provoked a discussion on whether these age limits still hold and if different limits should be used for white and black American children. It was recommended to use age limits of 7 years in white and 6 years in black girls [48]. However, since the pubertal onset has advanced but not the timing of menarche, the question can be addressed whether the cases of early puberty reflect a change in normal physiologic development or an abnormal puberty. This discussion is critical for the consideration of who needs to undergo diagnostic evaluation and therapeutic intervention. In 223 girls with breast development before the age of 8 years, it appeared that one third had seriously advanced bone age, and 12% had other endocrine disorders such as, among others, McCune-Albright syndrome, adrenal hyperplasia and growth hormone deficiency [49]. These data are very important and show that early breast development between the ages of 6 and 8 years is not necessarily a benign variant, and therefore still needs diagnostic evaluation.

The development of sex characteristics in central precocious puberty is the result of a too early start of the GnRH pulse generator. Endocrine evaluation shows pubertal levels of gonadotropins and sex steroids with the day night rhythm of LH characteristic of puberty. Figure 1 shows the 24-hour LH patterns of girls with central precocious puberty showing a more pronounced pulsatile pattern for LH during the night. The endocrine difference with physiologic puberty is the exaggerated gonadotropin response to GnRH (fig. 2), especially for LH, while basal gonadotropin and sex steroid levels do not differ from children in a similar stage of puberty. Since progression of puberty is often advanced in girls with central precocious puberty (fig. 3), one may suggest that the faster progression of puberty and the increased gonadotropin response to GnRH are the result of a more rapid development of the GnRH pulse generator with a retarded equilibrium between

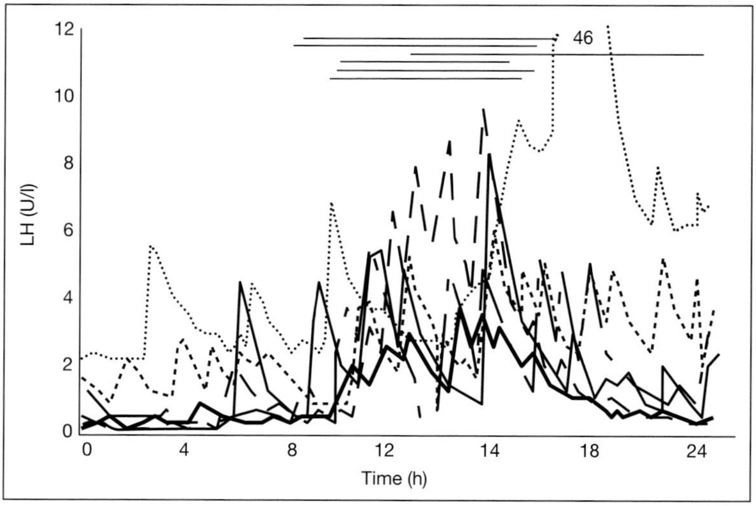

Fig. 1. 24-hour pulse patterns of LH in girls diagnosed to have idiopathic central precocious puberty. Nighttime levels show a distinct pulsatile secretion pattern with increased levels compared to daytime values. Sleep periods are indicated by horizontal lines. From Schroor et al [50].

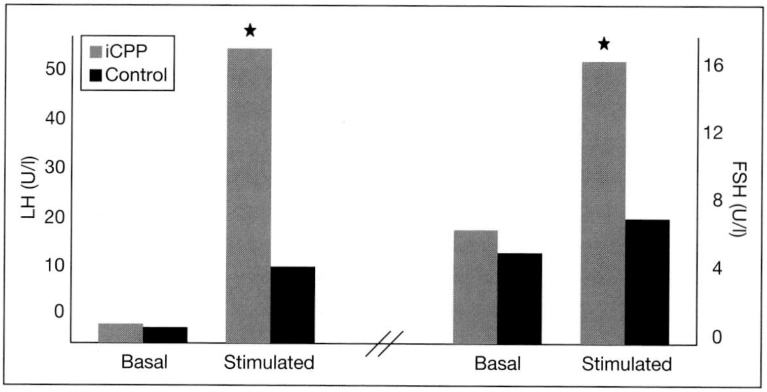

Fig. 2. Basal and GnRH (100 μg i.v.) stimulated levels of LH and FSH in 14 girls with idiopathic central precocious puberty and 21 controls in similar stages of puberty. Estradiol levels between the idiopathic central precocious puberty girls and controls did not differ significantly (idiopathic central precocious puberty 92.7 ± 23 (SD), controls 65.4 ± 13 pmol/l resp.). Basal levels of LH and FSH do not differ, while LH and FSH peak levels are significantly higher in the affected girls. iCPP = Idiopathic central precocious puberty.

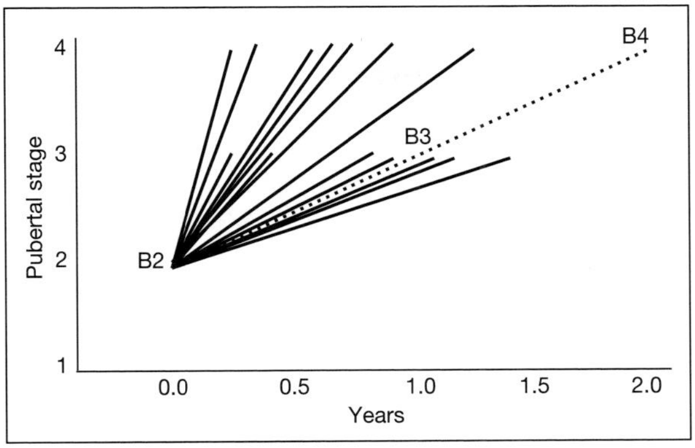

Fig. 3. Progression of puberty from B2 to B3 or B4 in girls with idiopathic central precocious puberty. The broken line indicates approximate mean progression, calculated from transversal data in healthy Dutch girls [51].

gonadal steroids and gonadotropin secretion. Treatment with GnRH analogues in order to suppress gonadotropin secretion will bring the patient temporarily in a prepubertal state, but will not postpone central pubertal development [50]. This means that central maturation continues under GnRH analogue treatment resulting in a full-blown resumption of the endocrine axis after discontinuation.

In The Netherlands, delayed puberty is defined as a start of puberty in boys later than the age of 13.8 years and in girls 12.7 years based on the 97th centile of puberty onset [51]. Boys with delayed puberty may suffer from isolation from their peers, less self-esteem and identity disorders [52]. Most of them will undergo spontaneous puberty, only later. From the physical point of view delayed puberty does not need to be treated medically. However, since increasing evidence is becoming available that these adolescent circumstances may compromise further development [53], one should consider treating adolescent boys with delayed puberty to support psychological development. Short courses of sex steroids are helpful for psychological reasons, but will not advance spontaneous puberty. Oxandrolone will only increase height velocity. Based on the individual problem, the pediatrician may consider either treatment with androgens or oxandrolone in a boy with delayed puberty.

It is unclear why more boys than girls present with delayed puberty. The distribution of timing of puberty can be skewed with an increased number of male individuals in the late onset range? Or is it that boys have more problems related to late development than girls? This last option is most conceivable, since boys enter puberty at a later time than girls and sex characteristics such as increased height velocity, virilization and changing behavior do not occur before the second half of puberty.

Schroor and coworkers observed that in boys with late onset of puberty the progression through the pubertal stages is not retarded. A similar progression as in normal-timed puberty can be observed [54]. Subsequently, short courses of sex steroids are helpful with respect to psychological interference, but will not advance spontaneous puberty, while oxandrolone will only increase height velocity [55]. This benign variant of pubertal development can be cumbersome for the male adolescent and therefore intervention is very helpful.

References

1 Kaplan SL, Grumbach MM: Pituitary and placental gonadotrophins and sex steroids in the human and sub-human primate fetus. Clin Endocrinol Metab 1978;7:487–511.

2 Conte FA, Grumbach MM, Kaplan SL, Reiter EO: Correlation of luteinizing hormone-releasing factor-induced luteinizing hormone and follicle-stimulating hormone release from infancy to 19 years with the changing pattern of gonadotropin secretion in agonadal patients: Relation to the restraint of puberty. J Clin Endocrinol Metab 1980;50:163–168.

3 Kaplan SL, Grumbach MM, Aubert ML: The ontogenesis of pituitary hormones and hypothalamic factors in the human fetus: Maturation of central nervous system regulation of anterior pituitary function. Recent Prog Horm Res 1976;32:161–243.

4 Stanhope R, Pringle PJ, Brook CG: The mechanism of the adolescent growth spurt induced by low dose pulsatile GnRH treatment. Clin Endocrinol (Oxf) 1988;28:83–91.

5 Klein KO, Baron J, Barnes KM, Pescovitz OH, Cutler GB Jr: Use of an ultrasensitive recombinant cell bioassay to determine estrogen levels in girls with precocious puberty treated with a luteinizing hormone-releasing hormone agonist. J Clin Endocrinol Metab 1998;83:2387–2389.

6 Tanner JM: A History of the Study of Human Growth. University Press, Cambridge, 2004.

7 Muinck Keizer de SM, Mul D: Trends in pubertal development in Europe. Hum Reprod Update 2001;7:287–291.

8 Herman-Giddens ME, Slora EJ, Wasserman RC, Bourdony CJ, Bhapkar MV, Koch GG, et al: Secondary sexual characteristics and menses in young girls seen in office practice: A study from the Pediatric Research in Office Settings network. Pediatrics 1997;99:505–512.

9 Herman-Giddens ME, Wang L, Koch G: Secondary sexual characteristics in boys: Estimates from the national health and nutrition examination survey III, 1988–1994. Arch Pediatr Adolesc Med 2001;155:1022–1028.

10 Kaplowitz PB, Slora EJ, Wasserman RC, Pedlow SE, Herman-Giddens ME: Earlier onset of puberty in girls: Relation to increased body mass index and race. Pediatrics 2001;108:347–353.

11 Themmen APN, Huhtaniemi IT: Mutations of gonadotropins and gonadotropin receptors: Elucidating the physiology and pathophysiology of pituitary-gonadal function. Endocr Rev 2000;21:551–583.

12 Karges B: Molecular genetics of isolated hypogonadotropic hypogonadism and Kallmann syndrome. Abnormalities in puberty: Scientific and clinical advances. Endocr Dev. Basel, Karger, 2005, vol 8, pp 67–80.

13 Weiss J, Axelrod L, Whitcomb RW, Harris PE, Crowley WF, Jameson JL: Hypogonadism caused by a single amino acid substitution in the beta subunit of luteinizing hormone. N Engl J Med 1992;326:179–183.

14 Nilsson C, Pettersson K, Millar RP, Coerver KA, Matzuk MM, Huhtaniemi IT: Worldwide frequency of a common genetic variant of luteinizing hormone: An international collaborative research. International Collaborative Research Group. Fertil Steril 1997;67:998–1004.

15 Raivio T, Huhtaniemi I, Anttila R, Siimes MA, Hagenas L, Nilsson C, et al: The role of luteinizing hormone-beta gene polymorphism in the onset and progression of puberty in healthy boys. J Clin Endocrinol Metab 1996;81:3278–3282.

16 Ramanujam LN, Liao WX, Roy AC, Ng SC: Association of molecular variants of luteinizing hormone with male infertility. Hum Reprod 2000;15:925–928.
17 Liao WX, Roy AC, Chan C, Arulkumaran S, Ratnam SS: A new molecular variant of luteinizing hormone associated with female infertility. Fertil Steril 1998;69:102–106.
18 Lindstedt G, Nystrom E, Matthews C, Ernest I, Janson PO, Chatterjee K: Follitropin (FSH) deficiency in an infertile male due to FSH-beta gene mutation. A syndrome of normal puberty and virilization but underdeveloped testicles with azoospermia, low FSH but high lutropin and normal serum testosterone concentrations. Clin Chem Lab Med 1998;36:663–665.
19 Layman LC, Lee EJ, Peak DB, Namnoum AB, Vu KV, van Lingen BL, et al: Delayed puberty and hypogonadism caused by mutations in the follicle-stimulating hormone beta-subunit gene. N Engl J Med 1997;337:607–611.
20 Kremer H, Martens JW, van Reen M, Verhoef-Post M, Wit JM, Otten BJ, et al: A limited repertoire of mutations of the luteinizing hormone (LH) receptor gene in familial and sporadic patients with male LH-independent precocious puberty. J Clin Endocrinol Metab 1999;84:1136–1140.
21 Toledo SP: Leydig cell hypoplasia leading to two different phenotypes: Male pseudohermaphroditism and primary hypogonadism not associated with this. Clin Endocrinol (Oxf) 1992;36:521–522.
22 Aittomaki K, Herva R, Stenman UH, Juntunen K, Ylostalo P, Hovatta O, et al: Clinical features of primary ovarian failure caused by a point mutation in the follicle-stimulating hormone receptor gene. J Clin Endocrinol Metab 1996;81:3722–3726.
23 Tapanainen JS, Aittomaki K, Min J, Vaskivuo T, Huhtaniemi IT: Men homozygous for an inactivating mutation of the follicle-stimulating hormone (FSH) receptor gene present variable suppression of spermatogenesis and fertility. Nat Genet 1997;15:205–206.
24 Gromoll J, Simoni M, Nieschlag E: An activating mutation of the follicle-stimulating hormone receptor autonomously sustains spermatogenesis in a hypophysectomized man. J Clin Endocrinol Metab 1996;81:1367–1370.
25 Seminara SB, Hayes FJ, Crowley WF Jr: Gonadotropin-releasing hormone deficiency in the human (idiopathic hypogonadotropic hypogonadism and Kallmann's syndrome): Pathophysiological and genetic considerations. Endocr Rev 1998;19:521–539.
26 Dode C, Levilliers J, Dupont JM, De Paepe A, Le Du N, Soussi-Yanicostas N, et al: Loss-of-function mutations in FGFR1 cause autosomal dominant Kallmann syndrome. Nat Genet 2003; 33:463–465.
27 Seminara SB, Messager S, Chatzidaki EE, Thresher RR, Acierno JS Jr, Shagoury JK, et al: The GPR54 gene as a regulator of puberty. N Engl J Med 2003;349:1614–1627.
28 Beranova M, Oliveira LM, Bedecarrats GY, Schipani E, Vallejo M, Ammini AC, et al: Prevalence, phenotypic spectrum, and modes of inheritance of gonadotropin-releasing hormone receptor mutations in idiopathic hypogonadotropic hypogonadism. J Clin Endocrinol Metab 2001;86: 1580–1588.
29 Frisch RE, Revelle R: Height and weight at menarche and a hypothesis of menarche. Arch Dis Child 1971;46:695–701.
30 Ruf KB: How does the brain control the process of puberty? Z Neurol 1973;204:96–105.
31 Cheung CC, Thornton JE, Nurani SD, Clifton DK, Steiner RA: A reassessment of leptin's role in triggering the onset of puberty in the rat and mouse. Neuroendocrinology 2001;74:12–21.
32 Barker DJ: Developmental origins of adult health and disease. J Epidemiol Community Health 2004;58:114–115.
33 Ibanez L, de Zegher F, Potau N: Premature pubarche, ovarian hyperandrogenism, hyperinsulinism and the polycystic ovary syndrome: From a complex constellation to a simple sequence of prenatal onset. J Endocrinol Invest 1998;21:558–566.
34 Ibanez L, Ferrer A, Marcos MV, Hierro FR, de Zegher F: Early puberty: Rapid progression and reduced final height in girls with low birth weight. Pediatrics 2000;106:E72.
35 Delemarre-van de Waal HA, van Coeverden SC, Engelbregt MT: Factors affecting onset of puberty. Horm Res 2002;57(suppl 2):15–18.
36 Francois I, de Zegher F, Spiessens C, D'Hooghe T, Vanderschueren D: Low birth weight and subsequent male subfertility. Pediatr Res 1997;42:899–901.
37 Ibanez L, Potau N, de Zegher F: Ovarian hyporesponsiveness to follicle stimulating hormone in adolescent girls born small for gestational age. J Clin Endocrinol Metab 2000;85:2624–2626.

38 Engelbregt MJ, Houdijk ME, Popp-Snijders C, Delemarre-van de Waal HA: The effects of intrauterine growth retardation and postnatal undernutrition on onset of puberty in male and female rats. Pediatr Res 2000;48:803–807.
39 Engelbregt MJ, van Weissenbruch MM, Popp-Snijders C, Delemarre-van de Waal HA: Delayed first cycle in intrauterine growth-retarded and postnatally undernourished female rats: Follicular growth and ovulation after stimulation with pregnant mare serum gonadotropin at first cycle. J Endocrinol 2002;173:297–304.
40 Ong KK, Potau N, Petry CJ, Jones R, Ness AR, Honour JW, et al: Opposing influences of prenatal and postnatal weight gain on adrenarche in normal boys and girls. J Clin Endocrinol Metab 2004;89:2647–2651.
41 Ong KK, Petry CJ, Emmett PM, Sandhu MS, Kiess W, Hales CN, et al: Insulin sensitivity and secretion in normal children related to size at birth, postnatal growth, and plasma insulin-like growth factor-I levels. Diabetologia 2004;47:1064–1070.
42 Proos LA, Hofvander Y, Tuvemo T: Menarcheal age and growth pattern of Indian girls adopted in Sweden. I. Menarcheal age. Acta Paediatr Scand 1991;80:852–858.
43 Oostdijk W, Yap YN, Doude van Troostwijk ML, Rekers-Mombarg LTM, Massa GG, Brand R, et al: The impact of early puberty on final height in foreign born adopted children in the Netherlands. Horm Res 2004;35:24–29.
44 Gulledge CC, Burow ME, McLachlan JA: Endocrine disruption in sexual differentiation and puberty. What do pseudohermaphroditic polar bears have to do with the practice of pediatrics? Pediatr Clin N Am 2001;48:1223–1240,x.
45 Krstevska-Konstantinova M, Charlier C, Craen M, Du CM, Heinrichs C, de Beaufort C, et al: Sexual precocity after immigration from developing countries to Belgium: Evidence of previous exposure to organochlorine pesticides. Hum Reprod 2001;16:1020–1026.
46 Skakkebaek NE: Testicular dysgenesis syndrome. Horm Res 2003;60(suppl 3):49.
47 Lebrethon MC, Bourguignon JP: Management of central isosexual precocity: Diagnosis, treatment, outcome. Curr Opin Pediatr 2000;12:394–399.
48 Kaplowitz PB, Oberfield SE: Reexamination of the age limit for defining when puberty is precocious in girls in the United States: Implications for evaluation and treatment. Drug and Therapeutics and Executive Committees of the Lawson Wilkins Pediatric Endocrine Society. Pediatrics 1999;104:936–941.
49 Midyett LK, Moore WV, Jacobson JD: Are pubertal changes in girls before age 8 benign? Pediatrics 2003;111:47–51.
50 Schroor EJ, van Weissenbruch MM, Delemarre-van de Waal HA: Long-term GnRH-agonist treatment does not postpone central development of the GnRH pulse generator in girls with idiopathic precocious puberty. J Clin Endocrinol Metab 1995;80:1696–1701.
51 Mul D, Fredriks AM, van Buuren S, Oostdijk W, Verloove-Vanhorick SP, Wit JM: Pubertal development in The Netherlands 1965–1997. Pediatr Res 2001;50:479–486.
52 Schwab J, Kulin HE, Susman EJ, Finkelstein JW, Chinchilli VM, Kunselman SJ, et al: The role of sex hormone replacement therapy on self-perceived competence in adolescents with delayed puberty. Child Dev 2001;72:1439–1450.
53 Huisman J, Bosch JD, Delemarre vd Waal HA: Personality development of adolescents with hypogonadotropic hypogonadism. Psychol Rep 1996;79:1123–1126.
54 Schroor EJ, Odink RJH, Delemarre-van de Waal HA: Is androgen treatment useful in constitutional delay of puberty and growth in boys? Horm Res 1992;37(suppl 4):243.
55 Schroor EJ, van Weissenbruch MM, Knibbe P, Delemarre-van de Waal HA: The effect of prolonged administration of an anabolic steroid (oxandrolone) on growth in boys with constitutionally delayed growth and puberty. Eur J Pediatr 1995;154:953–957.

Henriette A. Delemarre-van de Waal, MD
Professor in Pediatric Endocrinology, VU University Medical Center
PO Box 7057, NL–1007 MB Amsterdam (The Netherlands)
Tel. +31 20 440895, Fax +31 20 4442422, E-Mail H.Delemarre@vumc.nl

Delemarre-van de Waal HA (ed): Abnormalities in Puberty. Scientific and Clinical Advances.
Endocr Dev. Basel, Karger, 2005, vol 8, pp 15–33

Fetal Nutrition and Timing of Puberty

M.M. van Weissenbruch, M.J.T. Engelbregt, M.A. Veening, H.A. Delemarre-van de Waal

Department of Pediatrics, Research Institute for Clinical and Experimental Neurosciences, VU University Medical Center, Amsterdam, The Netherlands

Abstract

Over the last decade growing evidence has been documented on the relationship between intrauterine growth retardation (IUGR) and pubertal development indicating changes in timing and progression of puberty. These changes in pubertal development are part of a growing list of IUGR-related diseases, which includes type 2 diabetes mellitus, cardiovascular disease, short stature and polycystic ovary syndrome. The influence of IUGR on the mechanisms behind the onset of puberty is still elusive. In the absence of prospective studies on gonadotropin-releasing hormone pulse patterns in IUGR children, other markers of pubertal development such as age at menarche in girls and progression of puberty have been employed. We investigated pubertal development and DHEAS levels in children born small for gestational age (SGA) after third trimester growth retardation and children born appropriate for gestational age (AGA). A faster progression of puberty was found in girls but not in boys. DHEAS levels tended to be higher in SGA children than in AGA children. In animal studies using two rat models, growth and onset of puberty based on perinatal undernutrition were also investigated. In one model intrauterine growth retardation was induced by ligation of the uterine arteries (IUGR) at day 17 of gestation and in the other model postnatal food restriction (FR) was induced by increasing litter size after birth until weaning. In both models, the rats showed a persistent growth failure. Onset of puberty was defined by vaginal opening (VO) in female rats and by balanopreputial separation (BPS) in male rats. At onset of puberty IUGR and FR rats had a lower body weight compared to controls, indicating that no threshold for body weight is needed for the onset of puberty. In the IUGR female rats, the onset of puberty was delayed and in the FR female rats the onset of puberty was in time. In both IUGR and FR female rats VO and first cycle were uncoupled. In IUGR female rats, at VO, at first cycle and at the age of 6 months the ovaries showed a decline in number of follicles indicating that intrauterine malnutrition in the female rat has a permanent influence on the growth and development of follicles. In the FR female rats, at VO, the ovaries showed a normal number of follicles but an abnormal maturation pattern. At the time of first cycle and at the age of 6 months normalization in follicle growth pattern was observed. These findings suggest that postnatal undernutrition has a transient influence on follicle growth and development. In male rats, both models showed delayed onset of puberty and impaired testicular function, as shown by decreased testosterone levels. These data indicate that early malnutrition during different critical developmental time windows may result in different long-lasting effects on pubertal development in both humans and rats.

In 1989, reports suggested that the fetal environment, as reflected in birth size, was related to the risk of noncommunicable diseases in adult life. This led to the development of the fetal origins of adult disease paradigm, which resulted in a refocusing of research effort to investigate the lifelong consequences of perinatal influences on chronic diseases [1–9] and the function of neuroendocrine axes [10–13]. The principle that the nutritional, hormonal and metabolic environment afforded by the mother may permanently 'program' the structure and physiology of her offspring was established long ago. 'Programming' describes the process whereby a stimulus or an insult, at a sensitive or critical period of development, has lasting or lifelong significance [14, 15]. The essence of programming is based on the fact that changes of a system appear during a critical period when the system is plastic and sensitive to the environment. After the critical period, the changes remain due to loss of plasticity and fixed functional capacity.

The abundance of data on the short- and long-term diseases associated with IUGR contrasts with the scarcity of data on the transitional period including puberty. Although there is some evidence, it is not clear whether pubertal development is involved in this disregulation as well. However, based on a large body of evidence that the hypothalamic-pituitary-gonadotropin apparatus in the human fetus is functional by 50 days of gestation one can believe that also the maturational process of this endocrine unit can be influenced by 'programming', due to a poor intrauterine environment. Obviously, the regulatory systems involved in sexual physiology are plastic and can be permanently changed during sensitive time windows. The latter can be illustrated by the lifelong effect of early exposure to sex hormone on sexual physiology [16]. A female rat injected with testosterone propionate on the 5th day after birth develops normally until puberty, but fails to ovulate and does not show a normal pattern of female sexual behavior thereafter. Pituitary function is normal, but the release of gonadotropin-releasing hormone (GnRH) by the hypothalamus has been irreversibly altered from the cyclic female pattern of release into the tonic male pattern. If the same injection is given when the animal is 20 days old, it has not any effect on central regulation.

Puberty, defined as the achievement of the interactions between the neuroendocrine unit and the gonads, the hypothalamic-pituitary-gonadal axis, has in fact its origin in the fetal period, when this endocrine unit is already active. During infancy this endocrine unit becomes suppressed followed by a reactivation at the onset of puberty, characterized by activation of the hypothalamus and the pituitary initiating the sequence of changes leading to puberty. Of course, normal gonads are necessary for the completion of this maturational process leading to a fully mature state in adolescence.

Although the mechanisms behind the initiation of puberty have not been fully elucidated, a central regulation of the onset of puberty is most likely since agonadal children (e.g. children with Turner syndrome) show a normal biphasic pattern of GnRH secretion from the hypothalamus and a normal pattern of low levels of GnRH during the prepubertal years [17].

Pubarche (i.e. the appearance of pubic hair) is part of a broader definition of puberty and precedes GnRH reawakening. Pubarche is, however, related to adrenarche with increasing activity of adrenal androgens. Adrenarche does not influence the initiation of central pubertal development [18]. Nevertheless, an earlier and exaggerated adrenarche and pubarche has been linked with intrauterine growth retardation (IUGR) and pathology as well [19, 20].

Regarding a central, GnRH-mediated puberty there are studies that suggest an earlier onset in girls with IUGR as measured by age at menarche [21–23]. In contrast, others found barely any difference or even found an earlier onset of puberty in heavier newborns [24–26]. In the absence of prospective studies that compare nightly GnRH pulsatile patterns, it is not clear whether or not there is an earlier onset of puberty in IUGR girls. Data of pubertal development in boys born small for gestational age (SGA) are even scarcer.

Earlier onset of puberty has been reported in studies using markers of puberty (e.g. breast stage, peak height velocity and age at menarche) but these findings can be explained by a rapid progression of pubertal development rather than an early onset [22].

Earlier onset of puberty seems of clinical relevance since recent studies show that early menarche is associated with an increased risk of breast cancer [27]. In addition, earlier onset of puberty or rapid progression through puberty might also influence final adult height [28].

Most animal studies have investigated the impact of changes in maternal and fetal nutrition and blood flow on fetal growth, postnatal growth, growth of various organs and the development of the various endocrine axes. Data on long-term effects of growth retardation on the timing of puberty are lacking.

The purpose of this review is to describe the involvement of the maturational process of puberty in relation to fetal life, investigated in the human as well as in animal models. Furthermore, to draw some tentative conclusions and advance speculations, questions will be put forward and posed for future research.

Material and Methods

Human Study

Study Population

Twenty-four healthy boys and 29 healthy girls participated in the study which is part of a larger ongoing project in which endocrine and metabolic variables are studied in healthy children who live in the same catchment area in Amsterdam and surroundings [29]. All children were born at term. SGA was defined as birth weight (BW) < the 10th percentile corrected for gestational age (GA), gender and parity; appropriate for gestational age (AGA) as BW ≥ the 10th percentile, using Dutch references [30]. The children were examined twice. Mean age (± SD) in the SGA children at *first visit* was 9.1 ± 1.1 years and in the AGA children 9.0 ± 1.1 years. All children were prepubertal according to the criteria of Tanner [31]. Testicular volume was measured as the mean of both testicle volumes, using the Prader orchidometer. In boys the prepubertal stage (G1) was defined as a lack of spontaneous genital development with a testicular volume of <4 ml. In girls the prepubertal stage (B1) was defined as a lack of breast development. When the child had entered puberty, pubertal stage was expressed as the percentage of the calendar age the child was supposed to have corresponding to their pubertal stage (CA/pubertal age × 100%) according to the reference data of the Dutch nationwide study [32].

First Visit

Weight, and height were measured and the body mass index (BMI) was calculated. Target height (TH) was calculated from the parents' heights. Target height in boys was calculated as height father + (height mother + 13)/2 + 4.5 cm. Target height in girls was calculated as height mother + (height father – 13)/2 + 4.5 cm. Catch-up growth was defined as a height within 1.3 SD of the TH SD score (height SD score–TH SD score) [33]. A tape measure was used to measure waist and hip circumferences. Skin-fold thickness was measured with Harpenden skinfold calipers at the biceps, triceps, subscapular and suprailiac sites. Total body fat mass was calculated by the sum of the 4 sites in millimeters (mm). Bone age (BA) was determined on an X-ray of the left hand. Plasma testosterone in males, estradiol in females and dehydroepiandrosterone sulfate (DHEAS) were measured.

Follow-Up Visit

This second examination took place 2.5 years after the first visit. Physical examination, laboratory tests and determination of BA were identical to the first visit. Mean age in the SGA children at follow-up was 11.6 ± 1.0 years and in the AGA children 11.6 ± 1.1 years.

Analytical Methods

DHEAS, estradiol, and testosterone were measured by radioimmunoassay techniques. Luteinizing hormone (LH) and follicle-stimulating hormone (FSH) were measured by immunometric assay techniques.

Statistical Analysis

Statistical analysis was performed using the Statistical Package for Social Sciences (SPSS 9.0 software). Results are expressed as means ± SD. Differences between the SGA and AGA group were tested by χ^2 test for qualitative variables and Student's t test for quantitative variables.

Animal Study

IUGR Rats

In timed pregnant Wistar rats, IUGR was induced by bilateral ligation of the uterine artery on day 17 of gestation according to a modified method of Wigglesworth [34]. The pups were born spontaneously at day 21–22 and defined as IUGR if their weight on day 2 after birth was below 5.3 g, corresponding with −2 SDs of the mean of the weight of control pups born from sham-operated dams.

Food-Restricted Rats

Postnatal undernutrition was achieved by litter enlargement to 20 pups per mother from day 2 after birth until weaning (24 days). During lactation and postweaning, pups of all groups received a normal diet (20% protein).

Onset of Puberty

The onset of puberty was defined as the age (in days) at which vaginal opening (VO) in females or balanopreputial separation (BPS) occurred.

Body Mass Index

Body mass index was calculated by dividing body weight (g) by body length squared (cm^2). Body composition was measured with dual energy X-ray absorptiometry (DXA) (QRD 2000, Hologic, Waltham, Mass., USA) using the small animal software package [35].

Ovarian Histology and Follicle Counts at VO

At day of VO the rats were sacrificed. Both ovaries were dissected, weights were recorded and the ovaries were fixed in Bouin's fluid for 24 h and embedded in paraffin wax. Serial sections of 10 μm were stained with hematoxylin and eosin and in each fifth serial section the number of follicles was counted. Follicles were divided into primordial (type 1–3b), growing (type 4–5b) and antral (type 6–8) classes [36–38] and counted by use of a microscope.

Pregnant Mares Serum Gonadotropin (PMSG) Stimulation Test

Cyclic stages of the ovaries were studied by daily vaginal smears after VO. Two experimental protocols were set up for food-restricted (FR) rats. Study A was performed with controls (n = 11), IUGR rats (n = 9) and FR rats (n = 12) of the same age as controls in their first cycle. In study B, FR rats (n = 15) in their first cycle (i.e. 2 months later compared to the first cycle of controls) and age-matched controls (n = 9) were investigated. Study A, 50 IU PMSG (Sigma Chemicals, Colo., USA) was injected intraperitoneally in IUGR rats and control rats on diestrous of the first cycle, FR rats were injected 2 days after VO. Study B FR rats were injected on diestrous of their first cycle and compared with age-matched controls. Forty-two hours later, the rats were sacrificed.

Ovarian Histology and Follicle Counts at the Age of 6 Months

The procedure described above was repeated at the age of 6 months.

Testicular function

Testicular function tests were performed in control (n = 12), IUGR (n = 10) and FR rats (n = 16), which were sacrificed at BPS. Both testes were dissected and weights were recorded. Blood was collected via cardiac puncture and serum was stored at −20°C until assayed for testosterone and leptin.

Leydig Cell Counts

Leydig cells were measured according a previously described procedure [39] of the mouse Leydig cell assay (MLCA). After decapsulation, the testes were cut into small pieces and placed in 5 ml Gibco M199 + 0.1% BSA. After 10 min stirring for detaching the Leydig cells, the mixture was filtered through monodur polyamide gauze (mesh size 100 μm, Stokvis & Smits, IJmuiden, the Netherlands). The filtrate was centrifuged during 10 min at 150 *g*, the cells were resuspended in 3 ml fresh medium and counted in a Burker counting chamber.

Analytical Methods

Testosterone and leptin were measured by radioimmunoassay techniques.

Statistical Analysis

Data are expressed as mean ± SEM. Statistical analyses were performed using ANOVA, followed by Dunnett's test for multiple comparisons of the two treated groups with controls.

In the second experiment, the Student's t test was performed to compare the FR group at first cycle with controls. Differences were considered statistically significant when $p < 0.05$.

Results

Human Study [40]

Clinical Characteristics

Table 1 shows the clinical characteristics of the two groups, AGA and SGA, at birth and table 2 the characteristics at time of the two visits.

The change in BMI from birth to 11.5 years was higher in girls born SGA than in girls born AGA (6.2 ± 2.9 vs. 3.7 ± 3.0 kg/m^2; p = 0.05). BMI in SGA girls changed from 10.8 ± 0.9 at birth to 16.3 ± 2.6 kg/m^2 at 11.5 years, in AGA girls from 13.9 ± 0.8 to 17.4 ± 3.8 kg/m^2. This change in BMI was not different in boys born SGA compared to boys born AGA (5.4 ± 2.6 vs.4.6 ± 3.0 kg/m^2; p = 0.6). BMI in SGA boys changed from 11.7 ± 0.8 at birth to 15.1 ± 1.9 kg/m^2 at 11.5 years, in AGA boys from 13.0 ± 2.0 to 17.3 ± 3.2 kg/m^2.

Table 1. Clinical characteristics at birth

	AGA (n = 24)	SGA (n = 29)
At birth		
Gender (male/female)	12/12	12/17
Gestational age, days	278 ± 10	276 ± 10
Birth weight, g	3,471 ± 475	2,442 ± 279*
Birth length, cm	50.7 ± 2.3	46.9 ± 2.3*
Ponderal index, g/cm^3 × 100	26.6 ± 3.2	24.0 ± 2.5*

*p < 0.001 AGA vs. SGA.

Table 2. Clinical characteristics at first visit and at follow-up after 2.5 years in SGA and AGA children

	First visit		Second visit	
	AGA (n = 24)	SGA (n = 29)	AGA (n = 22)	SGA (n = 26)
Age, years	9.0 ± 1.1	9.1 ± 1.1	11.6 ± 1.1	11.6 ± 1.0
Body weight, kg	30.9 ± 5.5	29.5 ± 7.5	42.1 ± 9.7	41.0 ± 11.0
Height, cm	138.0 ± 6.2	135.2 ± 9.1	153.5 ± 9.3	150.9 ± 10.6
Height SDS-THSDS	−0.50 ± 0.8	−0.60 ± 0.8	−0.2 ± 1.1	−0.5 ± 0.9
BMI, kg/m^2	17.3 ± 3.4	15.8 ± 2.4	17.5 ± 2.6	17.2 ± 2.5
Waist-hip ratio	0.87 ± 0.04	0.87 ± 0.04	0.83 ± 0.03	0.83 ± 0.04
Total skin fold thickness, mm	30.7 ± 14.4	32.2 ± 14.2	33.9 ± 16.7	34.7 ± 13.6
Skeletal maturation (CA/BA)	1.1 ± 0.2	1.0 ± 0.2	1.1 ± 0.1	1.0 ± 0.1
Prepubertal	24	29	7	6
Pubertal	0	0	15	20

CA = Calendar age; BA = bone age.

Pubertal Development

At the first visit all children were prepubertal (table 2). DHEAS concentrations were significantly higher in SGA children than in AGA children (2.0 ± 1.1 vs. 1.3 ± 0.6 μmol/l; $p = 0.004$, after correction for chronological age $p = 0.003$).

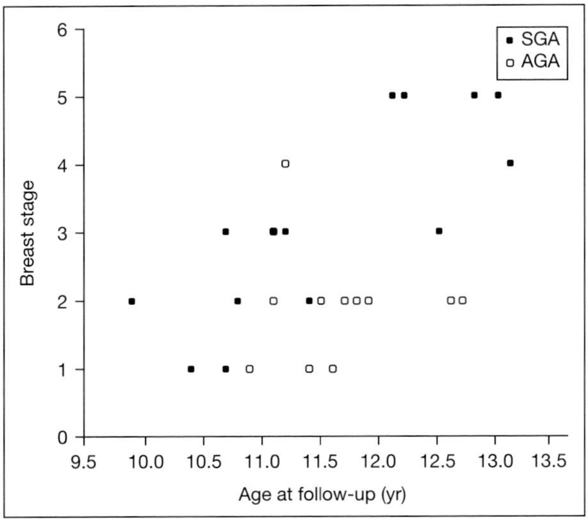

Fig. 1. Breast stage at follow-up in girls born SGA and girls born AGA.

At follow-up, 2.5 years later, 20 of 26 SGA children and 15 out of 22 AGA children were pubertal. CA/reference pubertal age for that stage × 100% was lower in SGA girls than in AGA girls (94.4 ± 7.1 vs. 106.4 ± 10.4; $p = 0.004$). However, CA/pubertal age × 100% was not different between SGA boys and AGA boys (104.7 ± 7.6 vs. 97.0 ± 8.4; $p = 0.1$). SGA girls have a more advanced breast stage at a certain calendar age than their AGA controls (fig. 1). Interestingly, 5 SGA children had reached a breast stage 4 or 5 within 2.5 years. At time of the study, 1 AGA girl (breast stage 4) and 4 SGA girls (all breast stage 5) had reached menarche. In boys no evident differences in genital stages between SGA and AGA were observed (fig. 2). DHEAS levels were higher in SGA children compared with AGA children (3.5 ± 1.8 vs. 2.5 ± 1.1 μmol/l; $p = 0.06$, after correction for chronological age $p = 0.07$).

Linear Growth

At the first visit, 5 SGA children (3 boys, 2 girls) did not show complete catch-up growth in height, defined as an actual height 1.3 SD or more below the THSDS [32]. Height in pubertal girls was similar in SGA and AGA children (156.0 ± 5.4 vs. 157.0 ± 7.0 cm; $p = 0.7$). The same was true for pubertal boys (153.3 ± 8.5 vs. 154.6 ± 11.6 cm; $p = 0.8$). Skeletal maturation, expressed as chronological age/bone age (CA/BA), was not different between SGA and AGA girls and between SGA and AGA boys at the first visit (girls: 0.8 ± 0.1

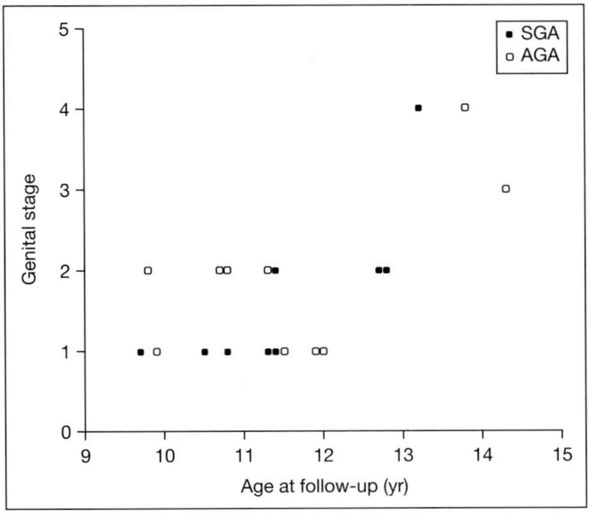

Fig. 2. Genital stage at follow-up in boys born SGA and boys born AGA.

vs. 0.8 ± 0.1; p = 0.3, boys: 0.8 ± 0.1 vs. 0.8 ± 0.1; p = 0.7) and at follow-up (girls: 1.0 ± 0.1 vs. 1.1 ± 0.1; p = 0.1, boys: 1.1 ± 0.2 vs. 1.1 ± 0.1; p = 0.6).

Animal Study [41–43]

Timing of Puberty [41]

In female IUGR rats (n = 37) compared to controls (n = 23) the age at VO was delayed (37.4 ± 2.7 vs. 36.1 ± 1.5 days; p < 0.04), but not in female FR rats (n = 18) (36.5 ± 2.2 vs. 36.1 ± 1.5 days). In male IUGR (n = 26) and FR (n = 20) rats the age at BPS was delayed compared to controls: IUGR: 48.1 ± 1.9 days (p < 0.0001), FR: 50.4 ± 2.9 days p < 0.0001) and controls (n = 30): 45.8 ± 1.4 days.

Weight and Body Composition at Onset of Puberty [41, 43]

Weight at onset of puberty in female IUGR and FR rats, was lower compared to controls: IUGR 106.1 ± 13.1 g (p < 0.001), FR 85.3 ± 7.6 g (p < 0.0001) and controls 116.9 ± 9.3 g. In male rats weight at onset of puberty did not differ between IUGR and controls (194.5 ± 20.0 vs. 201.7 ± 16.8 g) but was lower in FR rats (175.6 ± 17.5 g, p < 0.0001).

At onset of puberty in IUGR female and male rats no differences were found in body mass index, body composition and leptin levels compared to controls.

Table 3. Number of follicles at VO

	Controls (n = 8)	IUGR (n = 13)	FR (n = 9)
Primordial	45 ± 5	12 ± 1**	66 ± 10*
Growing	64 ± 8	36 ± 3**	79 ± 6
Antral	38 ± 7	29 ± 3	37 ± 3
Corpora lutea (CL)	6 ± 1	0***	0***
Antral + CL	44 ± 7	29 ± 3*	37 ± 3
Total number	152 ± 15	77 ± 5**	182 ± 16

Values are expressed as mean ±SEM. *p < 0.05, **p < 0.01, ***p < 0.001, compared with controls.

In contrast to IUGR rats, FR female rats compared to controls had a lower BMI (0.4038 ± 0.025 vs. 0.4774 ± 0.027 g/cm^2; p < 0.01), percentage of fat (9.67 ± 1.2 vs. 12.39 ± 1.6%; p < 0.01), and serum leptin levels (1.4 ± 0.4 ng/ml; p < 0.05) at VO. FR male rats compared to controls had a lower percentage of fat (10.54 ± 1.7 vs.12.15 ± 1.9%; p < 0.05) and serum leptin concentration (2.1 ± 0.7 vs. 3.0 ± 1.0 ng/ml; p < 0.05) at BPS.

Ovarian Development at Onset of Puberty

At onset of puberty the ovaries of IUGR rats contained a lower number of primordial and growing and total number of follicles compared to controls (all p < 0.01). The number of antral follicles in the ovaries did not differ between IUGR rats and controls but in contrast to the controls, no corpora lutea (CL) were observed in the ovaries of the IUGR rats (p < 0.001).

The ovaries of the FR rats had a higher number of primordial follicles (p < 0.05) and also in the FR rats no CL were observed (p < 0.001) (table 3). Figure 3 shows ovaries of a control, an IUGR and an FR rat with different stages of developing follicles at onset of puberty. Note the absence of corpora lutea in the ovary of the IUGR and FR rat.

With respect to first cycle it was obvious that in contrast to controls in which vaginal opening and first cycle took place on the same day, in IUGR rats VO and first cycle were uncoupled. VO was delayed (p < 0.05) and the first cycle was even further delayed (p < 0.01). Body weight in IUGR rats was lower (p < 0.05) at VO, but at first cycle and after stimulation with 50 IU PMSG in the first cycle, BW was not different compared to controls. The number of primordial (p < 0.05), growing (p < 0.01), antral follicles (p < 0.01) and the total number of follicles (p < 0.01) were lower compared to controls

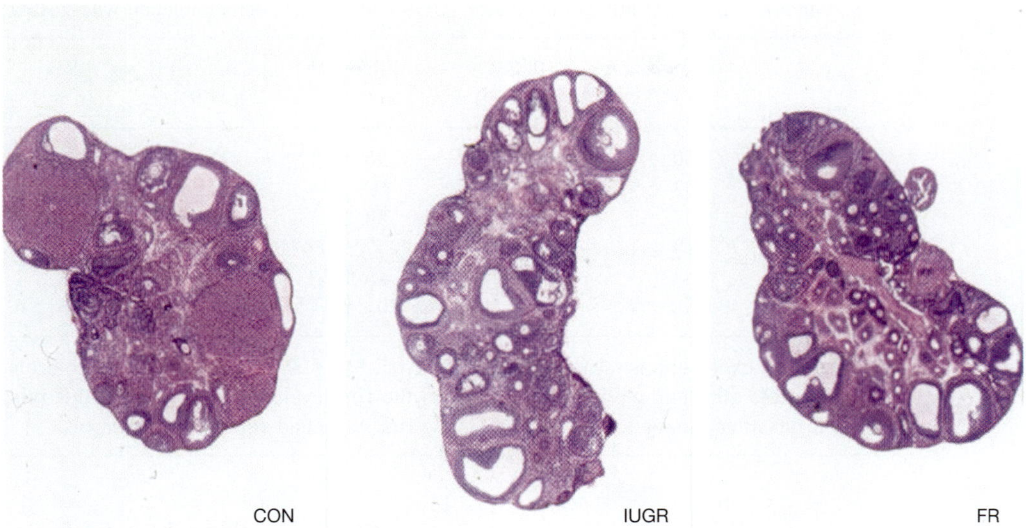

Fig. 3. Ovaries of a control, an IUGR and FR rat with different stages of developing follicles at onset of puberty. Note the absence of corpora lutea in the ovary of the IUGR and FR rat.

after stimulation with 50 IU PMSG at first cycle. The number of CL was similar and reflected superovulation (table 4).

In the FR rats, VO occurred at the same time as in the controls but at a lower BW ($p < 0.01$). First cycle was much delayed ($p < 0.01$), at which BW was higher ($p < 0.01$) compared to controls at first cycle. Based on the differences in weight and age between FR rats and controls at first cycle two studies were performed. In study A, control rats at first cycle and age-matched FR rats were investigated. In study B, FR rats at first cycle and age-matched control rats were examined. PMSG stimulation in the FR rats of study A resulted in a higher total number of follicles ($p < 0.05$), represented by a higher number of primordial follicles ($p < 0.01$) and a lower number of antral follicles ($p < 0.05$) and corpora lutea ($p < 0.01$) compared to controls. The total number of follicles in the ovaries of the FR rats of study B did not differ from the age-matched controls after PMSG stimulation at first cycle, nor was the number of follicles in the different classes (table 4).

Ovarian Development at the Age of Six Months

At the age of 6 months, the IUGR and FR rats both showed similar ovulation rate compared to controls. No differences were found in the number of follicles in the different classes between the FR rats and controls. The IUGR

Table 4. Number of follicles in control, IUGR and FR rats after stimulation with PMSG

	Controls A (n = 11)	IUGR (n = 9)	FRA (n = 12)	Controls B (n = 9)	FRB (n = 15)
Primordial	60 ± 7	31 ± 4*	96 ± 11**	41 ± 3	39 ± 4
Growing	53 ± 3	36 ± 3**	59 ± 4	75 ± 4	65 ± 3
Antral	37 ± 2	27 ± 2**	38 ± 2	31 ± 1	30 ± 1
CL	18 ± 1	18 ± 1	7 ± 0.4**	23 ± 1	21 ± 1
Antral + CL	54 ± 3	45 ± 2*	46 ± 3*	54 ± 1	51 ± 1
Total	168 ± 9	113 ± 7**	201 ± 14*	170 ± 6	156 ± 6

Values are expressed as mean ±SEM. *$p < 0.05$, **$p < 0.01$, compared with controls. A = Controls after stimulation with PMSG in the first cycle and age-matched FR rats; B = FR rats after stimulation with PMSG in the first cycle and age-matched controls.

rats, primordial ($p < 0.01$), growing ($p < 0.05$) and total number of follicles ($p < 0.01$) were lower compared to the control rats (table 5).

Testicular Development at Onset of Puberty

Although male IUGR rats had a delayed BPS ($p < 0.01$), at that time body weight was not different between IUGR rats and controls, nor was the serum leptin level. The number of Leydig cells ($\times 10^6$/testis at BPS) of IUGR rats was not different (5.0 ± 0.3 vs. 5.7 ± 0.3) but the testosterone levels were lower compared to controls (3.3 ± 0.6 vs. 5.9 ± 0.8 nmol/l; $p < 0.05$).

Also in the FR rats, BPS was delayed compared to controls ($p < 0.01$) and was accompanied by a lower body weight ($p < 0.05$). At that time the number of Leydig cells ($\times 10^6$/testis at BPS) (3.6 ± 0.3 vs. 5.7 ± 0.3; $p < 0.01$) serum testosterone (3.6 ± 0.6 vs. 5.9 ± 0.8 nmol/l; $p < 0.05$) and leptin levels (2.3 ± 0.2 vs. 3.4 ± 0.4 ng/ml; $p < 0.05$) were lower.

Discussion

The initiation and progression of puberty is complex and many factors have been identified which influence GnRH production or secretion either directly or indirectly. It has been suggested that this process controlled by genetic factors is not only mediated by environmental circumstances that originate through nutrition during infancy and childhood [44–46] but also during fetal life.

Recent studies indicate that the onset of puberty and menarche are linked to a combination of intrauterine and postnatal growth patterns [22, 47]. However, in the absence of prospective studies that compare nightly GnRH

Table 5. Number of follicles in control, IUGR and FR rats at the age of 6 months

	Controls (n = 6)	IUGR (n = 4)	FR (n = 5)
Primordial	45 ± 4	23 ± 4**	41 ± 2
Growing	53 ± 4	33 ± 4*	40 ± 5
Antral	34 ± 2	31 ± 3	33 ± 4
CL	7 ± 0.3	7 ± 0.7	6 ± 0.5
Antral + CL	41 ± 2	38 ± 3	39 ± 5
Total	139 ± 8	94 ± 9**	120 ± 9

Values are expressed as mean ±SEM. *$p < 0.05$, **$p < 0.01$, compared with controls.

pulsatile patterns, it remains unclear whether or not the onset of puberty is influenced by early growth. Studies so far have used markers of puberty that do not reflect the actual onset of central puberty. Therefore the findings described above can be explained by a rapid progression of pubertal development rather than an early onset.

Also, in the present study SGA girls who suffered from third trimester intrauterine growth retardation show a faster progression of pubertal development compared to AGA girls and the Dutch population [48]. Since current BMI and total skinfold thickness between SGA and AGA pubertal girls were similar but SGA girls had a higher increment in BMI from birth to 11.5 years, it can be suggested that the progression through puberty depends on a certain increase in body size rather than on the achievement of a certain body weight. A rapid progression to menarche in girls born SGA may compromise final adult height [28]. However, we did not observe an acceleration of skeletal maturation in SGA girls.

SGA and AGA boys showed no differences in pubertal stage at a certain calendar age. Previous studies in boys showed a positive relationship between age at onset of puberty and BMI [49]. In our study, current BMI and change in BMI from birth to 11.5 years in SGA boys were comparable to AGA boys. CA/PA × 100%, however, was >100 in SGA boys indicating that a certain pubertal stage was reached relatively late for their calendar age.

Animal studies also show a delayed onset of puberty in IUGR male rats [41]. The clinical relevance of such delay is not known yet. However, an association between male gonadal dysfunction and severely reduced fetal growth has been long recognized [50, 51]. Recently, Francois et al. [52] demonstrated that unexplained male subfertility is associated with low birth weight.

In the present study, higher DHEAS levels are found in SGA in comparison with AGA children. Ibanez et al. [53] previously demonstrated elevated DHEAS levels in asymptomatic nonobese, postmenarcheal girls born small for gestational age. In addition, they showed that minor fetal growth reduction appears to be associated with amplified adrenarche, whereas more pronounced prenatal growth restriction seems to precede functional ovarian hyperandrogenism during adolescence [19]. To study the prevalence of polycystic ovary syndrome (PCO) and subfertility in girls in the present study, longer follow-up is needed.

The clinical relevance of an exaggerated adrenarche levels in SGA boys is yet uncertain.

Overall the present data do support the concept that low birth weight as a consequence of intrauterine malnutrition has long-lasting effects on pubertal development as well as adrenal function.

The present studies in the IUGR and FR rat models focused on growth and timing of puberty in terms of structure and function of the gonads of both sexes.

The lower body weight at onset of puberty in IUGR and FR rats compared to controls, indicate that no threshold for body weight is needed for the onset of puberty. The differences in body mass index, body composition and serum leptin levels between the two rat models at that time also do suggest that onset of puberty in the rat is not dependent on a certain percentage of body fat or a certain threshold of leptin levels. On the other hand, it has to be questioned if these metabolic disturbances are at least in part responsible for the impaired sexual maturation in both male and female rats.

Further signs of impaired sexual maturation observed in IUGR and FR female rats were that VO and first cycle were uncoupled. In the IUGR female rat the delayed VO is explained by the lower number of developing follicles reaching appropriate estrogen levels at a later moment to obtain VO. The impaired follicle growth in IUGR rats may be the result of inadequate central stimulation since a similar ovulation rate compared to controls was observed after stimulation with exogenous PMSG. However, at the age of 6 months still a lower number of primordial and growing follicles and so total number of follicles but a similar spontaneous ovulation rate was observed compared to controls. These observations do suggest that intrauterine undernutrition in the female rat has a permanent influence on follicle growth and development.

In this view, we should consider that intrauterine growth retardation in the IUGR rat model takes place during a period of germ cell increment which may cause a permanent prenatal effect on the number of follicles. One may argue that these findings in the IUGR female rat are comparable in part with the second trimester undernutrition in humans. The resulting lower number of follicles may play a role in one of the origins of premature ovarian failure (POF) [54].

In the FR female rat, onset of puberty was associated with a higher number of growing follicles secreting sufficient estrogen to obtain VO in time. This impaired follicle growth and anovulation together with the decreased ovulation rate after exogenous PMSG stimulation around VO cannot differentiate between central and ovarian dysregulation. The observed normalization in follicle growth at time of first cycle after stimulation does suggest that postnatal undernutrition in the female rat has a transient influence on follicle growth and development. This was confirmed by the experiment at the age of six months showing a similar ovulation rate and follicle growth pattern.

The statement that oocyte and follicle maturation in the female rat occur after birth whereas in the human similar processes take place during fetal life is based on the finding of Oieda et al. [55] that follicle maturation is accompanied by comparable increments in FSH levels in the infantile female rat and the fetal human female.

Growth retardation after birth in the female rat may therefore be, at least partially, comparable with third-trimester IUGR in the human female. In the human female associations have been found between IUGR, insulin resistance and PCO [56–58]. In analogy with our findings in the rat, the prevalence of PCO is dependent on age among women: its presence is significantly higher among women at ages younger than 35 than among older women [59]. When PCO patients become older and hence cohort size decreases with age, a considerable number of these women restore their menstrual cycle regularity. The results in the FR female rat with respect to gonadal function support the findings of others that at least partially, the fundamental defect of PCO might be a consequence of (third trimester) intra-uterine growth retardation in the human female [19, 60].

Both IUGR and FR male rats showed a delayed onset of puberty. In the IUGR male rat, the low circulating testosterone levels at that time can be the result of either central dysregulation or dysfunction of the Leydig cells. Both have its origin during the intra-uterine period [55, 61–69]. Modification of GnRH neurons at the hypothalamic level may cause an impaired gonadotropin secretion leading to delayed puberty. On the other hand, we cannot exclude gonadal impairment since a disturbance in LH receptor production of the Leydig cell may cause in impaired sexual development as well [70].

The important phases of gonadal development in the male rat and the human male almost take place during the same periods [71, 72]. Therefore, IUGR in the male rat might be partially extrapolated to the human. As in the rat, intrauterine growth retardation in the human male may result in a delayed puberty and in fertility problems as a result of either central dysregulation or Leydig cell dysfunction. In general, the effect of intrauterine growth retardation on pubertal development in the human male has not been studied extensively. Francois et al. [52] noticed subfertility in boys born with a low birth weight.

They explained their results on central origin i.e. in terms of FSH insufficiency. FSH is important in regulating Sertoli cell multiplication. Therefore, early life modulation of FSH may decrease the number of Sertoli cells and so determines testicular size and sperm output in adulthood. Human studies with respect to the LH secretory pattern in relation to Leydig cell number and function have not been done yet. On the other hand, also in the human male one cannot exclude a gonadal impairment since a disturbance in LH receptor production of the Leydig cell itself may induce changes in sexual development.

In the male FR rat delayed onset of puberty was accompanied by low testosterone levels secreted by a lower number of Leydig cells. Postnatal undernutrition may influence the central regulation of the gonadal axis, since hypothalamic GnRH neurons and GnRH secretion continue to develop during that period [73]. On the other hand, postnatal undernutrition can also influence the process of adult Leydig cell maturation, which starts during that period [55].

Future Prospects

IUGR-related changes in puberty are of particular interest because of their relationship with chronic diseases in adulthood such as type 2 diabetes, polycystic ovary syndrome and short stature. Both animal and human studies have shown that insults during the perinatal period exert long-term effects on the metabolism of the offspring. One of the major problems in translating data from epidemiological studies to clinical practice is that is difficult to identify individuals who have been growth restricted in utero. Birth weight is only a crude index of early growth and reveals nothing about the success of a fetus at achieving its growth potential. Both the role of IUGR and mechanisms behind the initiation of puberty are still elusive. A key area of future research will be to identify markers of early growth restriction which may be of future diagnostic use as early predictors of adult disease. However, it must be kept in mind that there is a mutual dependency of genetic and environmental factors. In order to judge between them, research on pubertal development in monozygotic and dizygotic twins discordant for birth weight is of great interest.

References

1 Hales CN, Barker DJP, Clark PMS, Cox LJ, Fall C, Osmond C, Winter PD: Fetal and infant growth and impaired glucose tolerance at age 64. BMJ 1991;303:1019–1022.

2 Barker DJP, Gluckman PD, Godfrey KM, Harding JE, Owens JA, Robinson JS: Fetal nutrition and cardiovascular disease in adult life. Lancet 1993;341:938–941.

3 Gluckman PD, Cutfield W, Harding JE, Milner D, Jensen E, Woodhall S, Gallaher B, Bauer M, Breier BH: Metabolic consequences of intrauterine growth retardation. Horm Res 1996;48(suppl 1):11–16.

4 Gluckman PD, Harding JE: Fetal growth retardation: Underlying endocrine mechanisms and postnatal consequences. Acta Paediatr Suppl 1997;422:69–72.
5 Gluckman PD, Harding JE: The physiology and pathophysiology of intrauterine growth retardation. Horm Res 1997;48(suppl 1):11–16.
6 Godfrey KM, Barker DJP: Fetal nutrition and adult disease. Am J Clin Nutr 2000;71(suppl): 1344S–52S.
7 Eriksson JG, Forsen T, Tuomilehto J, Osmond C, Barker DJP: Early growth and coronary heart disease in later life: Longitudinal study. BMJ 2001;322:949–953.
8 Robinson R: The fetal origins of adult disease. BMJ 2001;322:375–376.
9 Harding JE: The nutritional basis of the fetal origins and adult disease. Int J Epidemiol 2001;30: 15–23.
10 Lucas A: Programming by early nutrition in man; in Bock GR, Whelen J (eds): The Childhood Environment and Adult Disease. Chichester, Wiley, 1991, pp 38–55.
11 Lucas A: Role of nutritional programming in determining adult morbidity. Arch Dis Child 1994;71:288–290.
12 Strauss RS: Effects of the intrauterine environment on childhood growth. Br Med Bull 1997;53: 81–95.
13 Barker DJP: Fetal nutrition and cardiovascular disease in later life. Br J Obstet Gynaecol 1996;103:814–817.
14 Zhernovaia NA: Maturation of the pituitary-gonadal system in girls born at term with low birth weight. Akusk Ginekol 1990;6:19–23.
15 Persson I, Ahlsson F, Wald U: Influence of perinatal factors on the onset of puberty in boys and girls: Implications for interpretation of link with risk of long-term diseases. Am J Epidemiol 1999;150:747–755.
16 Barraclough CA: Production of anovulatory, sterile rats by single injections of testosterone propionate. Endocrinology 1961;68:62–67.
17 Nathwani NC, Hindmarsh PC, Massarano AA, Brook CG: Gonadotrophin pulsatility in girls with the Turner syndrome: Modulation by exogenous sex steroids. Clin Endocrinol 1998;49:107–113.
18 Ibanez L, Virdis R, Potau N, Zampolli M, Ghizzoni L, Albisu MA, Carrascosa A, Bernasconi S, Vicens-Calvet E: Natural history of premature pubarche: An auxological study. J Clin Endocrinol Metab 1992;74:254–257.
19 Ibanez L, Potau N, Francois I, De Zegher F: Precocious pubarche, hyperinsulinism, and ovarian hyperandrogenism in girls: Relation to reduced fetal growth. J Clin Endocrinol Metab 1998;83: 3558–3562.
20 Ibanez L, De Zegher F, Potau N: Premature pubarche, ovarian hyperandrogenism, hyperinsulinism and the polycystic ovary syndrome: From a complex constellation to a simple sequence of prenatal onset. J Endocrinol Invest 1998;21:558–566.
21 Bhargava SK, Ramji S, Srivastava U, Sachdev HP, Kapani V, Datta V, Satyanarayana L: Growth and sexual maturation of low birth weight children: A 14 year follow up. Indian Pediatr 1995;32: 963–970.
22 Cooper C, kuh D, Egger P, Wadsworth M, Barker D: Childhood growth and age at menarche. Br J Obstet Gynaecol 1996:103:814–817.
23 Ibanez L, Ferrer A, Marcos MV, Hierro FR, De Zegher F: Early puberty: Rapid progression and reduced final height in girls with low birth weight. Pediatrics 2000;106:E72.
24 Albertsson-Wikland K, Karlberg J: Natural growth in children born small for gestational age with and without catch-up growth. Acta Paediatrica Suppl 1994;399:64–70.
25 Powls A, Botting N, Cooke RW, Pilling D, Marlow N: Growth impairment in very low birthweight children at 12 years: Correlation with perinatal and outcome variables. Arch Dis Child 1996;75:F152–F157.
26 Bacallao J, Amador M, Hermelo M: The relationship of birth weight with height at 14 and with the growing process. Nutrition 1996;12:250–254.
27 Stoll BA: Western diet, early puberty and breast cancer risk. Breast Cancer Res Tr 1998;187: 187–193.
28 Ibanez L, Ferrer A, Marcos MV: Early puberty: Rapid progression and reduced final height in girls with low birth weight. Paediatrics 2000;106:1–3.

29 Veening MA, van Weissenbruch MM, Delemarre-van de Waal HA: Glucose tolerance, insulin sensitivity, and insulin secretion in children born small for gestational age. J Clin Endocrinol Metab 2002;87:4657–4661.
30 Kloosterman GJ: Intrauterine growth and intrauterine growth curves. Ned Tijdschr Verloskd Gynaecol 1969;69:349–365.
31 Tanner JM: Growth and maturation during adolescence. Nutr Rev 1981;39:43–55.
32 Fredriks AM, van Buuren S, Burgmeijer RJF, Meulmeester JF, Beuker RJ, Brugman E, Roede MJ, Verloove-Vankorick P, Wit J: Continuing positive secular growth change in the Netherlands 1955–1997. Pediatr Res 2000;47:316–323.
33 Boukes FS, Merkx JAM, Rikken B, Huisman J: Opsporing, probleemverkenning, diagnostiek in de eerste lijn en criteria voor verwijzing; in De Muinck Keizer-Schrama SMPF (ed): Diagnostiek kleine lichaamslengte bij kinderen. Alphen aan den Rijn, Van Zuiden Communications, 1998.
34 Wigglesworth JS: Experimental growth retardation in the foetal rat. J Path Bact 1964;88:1–13.
35 Engelbregt MJT, Tromp AM, van Lingen A, Lips P, Popps-Snijders C, Delemarre-van de Waal HA: Validation of whole body DXA in young and adult rats. Horm Res 1999;51(suppl 2):P428.
36 Pedersen T, Peters H: Proposal for a classification of oocytes and follicles in the mouse ovary. J Reprod Fertil 1968;17:555–557.
37 Smith BJ, Plowchalk DR, Sipes IG, Mattison DR: Comparison of random and serial sections in assessment of ovarian toxicity. Reprod Toxicol 1991;5:379–383.
38 Bolon B, Bucci TJ, Warbritton AR, Chen JJ, Mattison DR, Heindel JJ: Differential follicle counts as a screen for chemically induced ovarian toxicity in mice: Results from continuous breeding bioassays. Fundam Appl Toxicol 1997;39:1–10.
39 Schroor EJ, van Weissenbruch MM, Engelbregt M, Martens F, Meurs JM, Wennink JM, Delemarre-van de Waal HA: Bioactivity of luteinizing hormone during normal puberty in girls and boys. Horm Res 1999;51:230–237.
40 Veening MA, van Weissenbruch MM, Roord JJ, Delemarre-van de Waal HA: Pubertal development in children born small for gestational age. J Pediatr Endocrinol Metab 2004;17:1497–1505.
41 Engelbregt MJ, Houdijk ME, Popp-Snijders C, Lips P, Delemarre-van de Waal HA: The effects of intra-uterine growth retardation and postnatal undernutrition on onset of puberty in male and female rats. Pediatr Res 2000;48:803–807.
42 Engelbregt MJ, van Weissenbruch MM, Popp-Snijders C, Delemarre-van de Waal HA: Delayed first cycle in intrauterine growth-retarded and postnatally undernourished female rats: Follicular growth and ovulation after stimulation with pregnant mare serum gonadotropin at first cycle. J Endocrinol 2002;173:297–304.
43 Engelbregt MJ, van Weissenbruch MM, Popp-Snijders C, Lips P, Delemarre-van de Waal HA: Body mass index, body composition, and leptin at onset of puberty in male and female rats after intrauterine growth retardation and after early postnatal food restriction. Pediatr Res 2001;50: 474–478.
44 Fredriks AM, van Buuren S, Burgmeijer RJF, Meulmeester JF, Beuker RJ, Brugman E, Roede MJ, Verloove-Vankorick P, Wit J: Continuing positive secular growth change in the Netherlands 1955–1997. Pediatr Res 2000;47:316–323.
45 Herman-Giddens ME, Slora EJ, Wasserman RC: Secondary sexual characteristics and menses in young girls seen in office practice: A study from the pediatric research in office settings network. Pediatrics 1997;99:505–512.
46 Huen KF, Leung SS, Lau JT, Cheung AY, Chiu MC: Secular trend in the sexual maturation of southern Chinese girls. Acta Paediatr 1997;86:1121–1124.
47 Adair LS: Size at birth predicts age at menarche. Pediatrics 2001;107:59–66.
48 Mul D, Fredriks M, van Buuren S, Oostdijk W, Verloove-Vanhorick SP, Wit JM: Pubertal development in The Netherlands 1965–1997. Pediatr Res 2001;50:479–486.
49 Vizmanos B, Marti-Henneberg C: Puberty begins with a characteristic subcutaneous body fat mass in each sex. Eur J Clin Nutr 2000;54:203–208.
50 Silver HK: Syndrome of congenital hemihypertrophy, shortness of stature and elevated urinary gonadotropin. Pediatrics 1953;12:368.
51 Angehrn V, Zachmann M, Prader A: Siver-Russell syndrome. Observations in 20 patients. Helv Paediatr Acta 1979;34:297–308.

52 Francois I, de Zegher F, Spiessens C, D'Hooghe T, Vanderschueren D: Low birth weight and subsequent male subfertility. Pediatr Res 1997;42:899–901.
53 Ibanez L, Potau N, Marcos MV, de Zegher F: Exaggerated adrenarche and hyperinsulinism in adolescent girls born small for gestational age. J Clin Endocrinol Metab 1999;84:4739–4741.
54 Hoek A, Schoemaker J, Drexhage HA: Premature ovarian failure and ovarian autoimmunity. Endocr Rev 1997;107–134.
55 Ojeda SR, Andrews WW, Advis JP, Smith White S: Recent advances in the endocrinology of puberty. Endocr Rev 1980;1:228–257.
56 Van der Meer M, Hompes PGA, de Boer JAM, Schats R, Schoemaker J: Cohort size rather than follicle-stimulating hormone threshold level determines ovarian sensitivity in polycystic ovary syndrome. J Clin Endocrinol Metab 1998;83:423–426.
57 Mason HD, Willis DS, Beard RW, Winston RM, Margara R, Franks S: Estradiol production by granulose cells of normal and polycystic ovaries: Relationship to menstrual cycle history and concentrations of gonadotropins and sex steroids in follicular fluid. J Clin Endocrinol Metab 1994;79:1355–1360.
58 Ibanez L, Valls C, Ferrer A, Marcos MV, Rodriquez-Hierro F, de Zegher F: Sensitization to insulin induces ovulation in nonobese adolescents with anovulatory hyperandrogenism. J Clin Endocrinol Metab 2001;86:3595–3598.
59 Koivunen R, Laatikkainen T, Tomas C, Huhtaniemi I, Tapanainen J, Martikainen H: The prevalence of polycystic ovaries in healthy women. Acta Obstet Gynecol Scand 1999;78:137–141.
60 Ibanez L, Potau N, Enriquez G, de Zegher F: Reduced uterine and ovarian size in adolescent girls small for gestational age. Pediatr Res 2000;47:575–577.
61 Benton L, Shan L, Hardy MP: Differentiation of adult Leydig cells. J Steroid Biochem Molec Biol 1995;53:61–68.
62 Ariyaratne HBS, Mason JI, Mendis-Handgama SMLC: Studies on the onset of Leydig precursor cell differentiation in the prepubertal rat testis. Biol Reprod 2000;63:165–171.
63 Mendis-Handagama SMLC, Risbridger GP, de Kretser DM: Morphometric analysis of the components of the neonatal and the adult rat testis interstitium. Int J Androl 1987;10:525–534.
64 Saez JM: Leydig cells: Endocrine, paracrine and autocrine regulation. Endocr Rev 1994;15:574–626.
65 Bartolussi M, Zanchetta R, Belvedere P, Columbo L: Sertoli and Leydig cell numbers and gonadotropin receptors in rat testis from birth to puberty. Cell Tissue Res 1990;260:185–191.
66 Tapanainen J, Kuopio T, Pelliniemi LJ, Huhtaniemi I: Rat testicular endogenous steroids and number of Leydig cells between the fetal period and sexual maturity. Biol Reprod 1984;31:1027–1035.
67 Kuopio T, Tapanainen J, Pelliniemi LJ, Huhtaniemi I: Developmental stages of fetal-type Leydig cells in prepubertal rats. Development 1989;107:213–220.
68 Kerr JB, Knell CM: The fate of fetal Leydig cells during the development of the fetal and postnatal rat testis. Development 1988;103:535–544.
69 Zirkin BR, Chen H, Luo L: Leydig cell steroidogenesis in aging rats. Exp Gerontol 1997;32:529–537.
70 Zirkin BR, Ewing LL: Leydig cell differentiation during maturation of the rat testis: A stereological study of cell number and ultrastructure. Anat Rec 1987;219:157–163.
71 Griffin JE, Wilson JD: 'The Testis'. Comprehensive Clinical Endocrinology, ed 3. St Louis, Mosby, 2002, pp 353–373.
72 Griffin JE, Wilson JD: Disorder of the Testes. Harrison's Principles of Internal Medicine, ed 15. New York, McGraw-Hill, 2001, pp 2143–2154.
73 Badger TM, Lynch EA, Fox PH: Effects of fasting on luteinizing hormone dynamics in the male rat. J Nutr 1985;115:788–797.

M.M. van Weissenbruch, MD, PhD
Department of Pediatrics, Research Institute for Clinical and
Experimental Neurosciences, VU University Medical Center
De Boelelaan 1117, NL–1081 HV Amsterdam (The Netherlands)
Tel. +31 0 20 4443014, Fax +31 0 20 4442422, E-Mail m.vanweissenbruch@vumc.nl

Delemarre-van de Waal HA (ed): Abnormalities in Puberty. Scientific and Clinical Advances.
Endocr Dev. Basel, Karger, 2005, vol 8, pp 34–53

Adrenal Function of Low-Birthweight Children

Ken Ong

Department of Paediatrics, University of Cambridge,
Addenbrooke's Hospital, Cambridge, UK

Abstract

During the neonatal period, increased stress due to infection or illness in low-birthweight infants may increase the importance of adequate adrenal cortisol secretion. Such low-birthweight infants often have transient cortisol insufficiency during the first few days of life, but then soon develop restored or even high cortisol levels. The pressure to enhance survival during this critical period could lead to either the programming of higher cortisol secretion, or the favorable selection of infants who are genetically predisposed to produce sufficient cortisol levels and activity. However, in long-term survivors of low birthweight, the maintenance of higher levels of cortisol secretion or action may contribute to increased hypertension and cardiovascular disease risk in later life. Similarly, low birthweight and subsequent rapid postnatal weight gain are associated with increased androgen secretion from the adrenal zona reticularis and this may contribute to disorders of hyperandrogenism and hyperinsulinemia before and after puberty. Precocious pubarche, the clinical manifestation of adrenal hyperandrogenism prepuberty, in girls is predictive of polycystic ovary syndrome, and is also associated with dyslipidemia, and increased central fat. In conclusion, long term consequences of low birthweight on both adrenal cortisol and adrenal androgen secretion could contribute to increased risks for the metabolic syndrome in later life.

Introduction

Impaired fetal growth has both short-term and long-term adverse consequences. In the short-term, low birthweight is associated with increased neonatal and infant mortality [1]. In the longer-term, low birthweight is associated with increased risk for the metabolic syndrome during adult life, including cardiovascular disease, type 2 diabetes and hypertension [2, 3]. The mechanisms that underlie these associations are still debated [4] and adrenal function, including both cortisol and androgen secretion, are candidates. Excess glucocorticoid exposure is a potential cause for poor antenatal growth, and there is increasing evidence for effects of low birthweight on adrenal glucocorticoid secretion, from the newborn to the elderly.

Glucocorticoid Exposure and Early Growth

Excess glucocorticoid exposure during early postnatal life has clear effects on limiting weight gain, growth in length, and long-term neurodevelopment [5]. A recent large, double-blind, placebo-controlled study in infants with severe respiratory distress syndrome showed that at age 8 years early postnatal dexamethasone therapy (0.25 mg/kg, intravenously every 12 hours for one week and then tapered) was associated with 1.6 cm shorter stature, 0.8 cm smaller head circumference, 6 points lower full IQ scores, poorer motor skills, and an increased frequency of clinically significant disabilities (39 vs. 22%) compared with controls [6].

Reinisch et al. [7] first described the link between low birthweight and antenatal glucocorticoid exposure, used to treat infertility and maintenance of pregnancy, and confirmed these effects on fetal growth in the mouse. Subsequent studies showed a dose-dependent effect of antenatal glucocorticoids on fetal growth restriction, and greater effects were seen in later pregnancy [8]. In sheep, a single maternal dose of betamethasone 0.5 mg/kg reduced birthweight by 11%, and three doses given weekly reduced birthweight by 19–25% [9]. The effects of more modest levels of antenatal glucocorticoid exposure on growth rates are not clear (discussed below), but could contribute to early suppression of adrenal function in the newborn [5].

Glucocorticoid Deficiency in the Low-Birthweight Newborn

Low circulating cortisol levels and adrenocortical insufficiency during the first few postnatal days are particularly seen among ill very-low-birthweight (VLBW: <1,500 g) premature infants, and are a cause of hypotension that is resistant to volume and inotrope support [10, 11]. A study of premature (<32 weeks' gestation), VLBW infants receiving ventilation support, showed that the majority had sub-optimal baseline cortisol levels (<414 nmol/l), and only 36–67% showed a response to increasing doses adrenocorticotrophic hormone (ACTH) [12]. Lower cortisol levels in the newborn predict worse short-term outcomes, including chronic lung disease and intraventricular hemorrhage

[12]. In another large study of 125 VLBW infants, lower cortisol levels even within the first few days of life predicted airway inflammation, patent ductus arteriosus, duration of oxygen therapy and chronic lung disease [13].

The defect is likely to be at the adrenal rather than pituitary level, as cortisol levels are low with normal or elevated ACTH levels [11], and cortisol responses to ACTH are poor [10, 12]. Contributory factors include degree of prematurity, as levels of cortisol, free cortisol and dehydroepiandrosterone sulfate (DHEAS) rise with increasing gestational age [14]. Elevated 11-deoxycortisol to cortisol ratios suggest that activity of 11β-hydroxylase, a key enzyme in cortisol biosynthesis, may be deficient in infants born <30 weeks' gestation [15]. Adrenocortical insufficiency may be particularly severe in VLBW infants of multiple pregnancies, possibly reflecting their more restrained antenatal growth [10]. Maternal glucocorticoid therapy for preterm labor may transiently suppress adrenocortical function in the newborn [16, 17]. High dose postnatal glucocorticoid therapy, to prevent or treat chronic lung disease, may also suppress endogenous basal and stimulated cortisol production, whether given intravenously or inhaled [14]. In some, particularly premature, low-birthweight infants persistence of adrenocortical insufficiency requires hydrocortisone replacement therapy [5].

However, adrenocortical insufficiency in the VLBW newborn is usually transient. Good recovery and even higher than average cortisol levels are seen by as early as postnatal day 14 [11, 16]. Such rapid adaptation of the hypothalamic-pituitary-adrenal axis to enhance cortisol secretion may be beneficial in the short-term, for example, by reducing chronic lung disease [13]. However, as seen following postnatal dexamethasone therapy [6], the continuation of higher glucocorticoid production could impair growth during early childhood. Even longer-term persistence of elevated cortisol levels might contribute to the fetal origins of adult disease links between low birthweight and metabolic disease risks.

Excess Glucocorticoid Secretion following Low Birthweight

The transition from glucocorticoid deficiency in the first few days of life to enhanced cortisol secretion, even within the neonatal period, is intriguing [11, 16]. The mechanism for this change is unknown, however there is growing evidence that this excess glucocorticoid secretion may continue into later life. It is well recognized that excess exogenous glucocorticoid administration or endogenous secretion (Cushing's syndrome) leads to central obesity, raised blood pressure and insulin resistance. Elevated cortisol levels following low birthweight could have more subtle effects, but have a significant contribution to the population risks for hypertension, type 2 diabetes and cardiovascular disease.

Animal Studies

The first reported association between low birthweight and higher cortisol levels was in female pigs [18]. At the age of 3 or 7 days, low-birthweight female pigs had 70 to 199% higher plasma cortisol levels, higher plasma cortisol binding globulin levels, greater cortisol responses to ACTH, and 46% larger adrenal gland weights (per kg birthweight) than in large birthweight pigs. Similar findings were reported in pigs at age 3 months (pre-pubertal juveniles), and at 12 months (young adults) [19]. In the latter study, low birthweight was also related to higher cortisol responses to ACTH at 3 months, but only in response to insulin induced hypoglycemia at 12 months, and it is unclear whether the programming of cortisol hyper-secretion is at the level of increased adrenal or pituitary response, or to both.

Fasting Cortisol Levels

Phillips et al. [20] reported the first population association between birthweight and plasma cortisol levels in 205 men from East Hertfordshire, UK. Fasting plasma cortisol levels fell progressively from 408 nmol/l in men with birthweights <5.5 lb (<2.50 kg) to 309 nmol/l with birthweights >9.5 lb (>4.31 kg). Furthermore, cortisol levels appeared to explain the low-birthweight associations with higher systolic blood pressure, fasting glucose levels, oral glucose intolerance, plasma triglyceride levels, and insulin resistance. Consistent associations were subsequently reported in each of three adult populations, from Adelaide, South Australia, Hertfordshire and Preston, UK [21]. In those studies each kilogram rise in birthweight was associated with a 23.9-mmol/l rise in plasma cortisol. These findings have also been confirmed in young adult populations from South Africa [22], and Hungary [23].

However, other studies have shown some inconsistencies. One smaller study of 52 young men and women found no differences in fasting plasma cortisol levels between low birthweight, premature appropriate birthweight, and full-term normal birthweight groups [24]. A further case control study of low birthweight vs. normal birthweight 12-year-old children found no difference in cortisol levels, despite a clear effect of birthweight on DHEAS levels [25]. The large ALSPAC study also found no association between birthweight and fasting cortisol levels in over 800 children at age 8 years, again despite clear effects of birthweight on adrenal androgen levels [26]. It is possible that differences in methodology could contribute to some of these discrepancies.

Methodological Considerations

A single blood measurement of cortisol or ACTH level provides a poor estimate of adrenal function because cortisol secretion is pulsatile. Three to four peaks of increasing amplitude occur overnight, and the last and highest peak may occur at anytime between 06.00 and 10.00 h [27]. Potential confounding factors that may raise fasting cortisol levels include longer duration of fasting, mild infection, and fear of venepuncture. Other methods for assessing cortisol secretion include 24-hour plasma cortisol profiles, and timed urine collections for measurement of total cortisol metabolites.

Higher urine cortisol levels have been reported in low-birthweight subjects [28]. However, again the results have not been consistent. In young adults, total urine cortisol metabolites were higher in both low-birthweight and premature groups, compared with normal birthweight full-term subjects; however, this finding was seen only in women but not in men [24]. In 190 children aged 9 years from Salisbury, UK, a quadratic or 'U-shaped' relationship between birthweight and total urinary cortisol metabolites was observed [29].

One study measured 24-hour plasma cortisol levels every 20 min in 83 elderly men and women. Mean cortisol levels between 07.30 and 09.00 h were slightly higher in subjects with lower birthweight ($p = 0.08$), but no birthweight associations were seen with other parameters of cortisol secretion, such as peak morning cortisol levels, regularity of pulses, and areas under the curve [30]. The authors therefore suggested that low birthweight might program adrenocortical sensitivity to stimulation rather than daily levels of cortisol secretion.

Dynamic Cortisol Responses

Stimulation with very low ACTH doses, such as one microgram, have been used to try to subjects with identify higher peak cortisol levels and increased adrenocortical sensitivity. Alternatively, a more important metabolic consequence of low birthweight could be the failure to suppress basal cortisol secretion, as seen in Cushing's syndrome.

Low-birthweight South African young adults had both 16% higher fasting cortisol levels and an identical 16% higher ACTH stimulated cortisol levels than normal birthweight controls [22]. Similarly, lower birthweight East Hertfordshire men aged 66–77 years had higher cortisol responses to ACTH, and also higher cortisol metabolites in a subsequent 24-hour urine collection [31]. In that study, the overnight suppression of cortisol levels following a very low dose of dexamethasone (0.25 mg) was unrelated to birthweight. However, the opposite findings of enhanced dexamethasone suppression of cortisol, but no difference in cortisol levels post-ACTH, were recently reported in low-birthweight Helsinki women aged 71 years [32].

In summary, it is still unclear whether the influence of low birthweight is largely on dynamic or resting cortisol secretion. In rats, programming of higher plasma cortisol levels by antenatal glucocorticoid exposure has been attributed to reduced negative feedback control of corticotrophin-releasing hormone and

ACTH, due to lower glucocorticoid receptor levels in the pituitary gland [33]. However, in low-birthweight humans there is yet no evidence for impaired central feedback by dexamethasone, but rather there is more data to support increased adrenal sensitivity to ACTH. While the mechanism of programming is unclear, cortisol hypersecretion does appear to contribute to increased metabolic syndrome risk in some low-birthweight populations. Both higher fasting and post-ACTH plasma cortisol levels have been shown to follow low birthweight and correlate with blood pressure, glucose levels and insulin resistance [31].

Antenatal Glucocorticoids and the Fetal Origins of Adult Disease

Variable findings in observation studies of birthweight and cortisol levels may indicate that only certain causes of low birthweight result in programming of subsequent higher cortisol secretion. Antenatal glucocorticoid exposure is a good candidate as it inhibits fetal growth, and in animal models can have long-term effects on metabolism, blood pressure and behaviour [33–36].

The Fetal Origins of Adult Disease studies in humans describe a continuous fall in rate of disease risk with increasing birthweight, throughout the whole range of birthweights [37]. Thus, if antenatal glucocorticoid exposure contributes to this link, it should be expected to influence the normal variation in birthweights. However, observations of current maternal glucocorticoid therapy, for the treatment of preterm labor, and less commonly for prevention of virilization in female offspring with congenital adrenal hyperplasia (CAH), report little effects on fetal growth.

Antenatal Steroids for Preterm Labor

Antenatal glucocorticoids are routinely given to women at risk of preterm delivery, before 32–34 weeks' gestation, in order to induce fetal alveolar surfactant secretion and improve lung function in the preterm newborn. In a recent Cochrane Library review antenatal glucocorticoid therapy reduced the incidence of respiratory distress syndrome (RDS) (odds ratio 0.53; 95% confidence interval 0.44–0.63), periventricular hemorrhage (0.29; 0.14–0.61), and neonatal mortality (0.60; 0.48–0.75) [38]. Betamethasone or dexamethasone are used, as these steroids cross the placenta into the fetus, at a total dose of 24 mg over 24–48 h [39].

While these doses have significant effects on maternal weight gain and blood pressure, follow-up studies show no effects on birthweight or childhood growth [40, 41]. Even in the absence of detectable growth suppression, children exposed to antenatal glucocorticoids may have higher blood pressures than those who were not exposed [42]. However, in that study the allocation of steroid treatment was non-random, and treatment-exposed children also had taller stature at age 14 years [43].

While only a single course is recommended, the maximal neonatal benefits of antenatal glucocorticoid therapy appear to wane after 7 days, and repeated weekly courses are often given up to 34 weeks' gestation [44]. There are some data suggesting that fetal growth may be affected by these higher doses. In a study of 477 singleton preterm infants, those exposed to ≥3 courses of antenatal steroids had a 9% reduction in birthweight and a 4% reduction in head circumference [45]. By 3 years of age, these children had shown appropriate catch-up growth. A review of 236 Chinese singleton pregnancies also found that exposure to ≥4 courses of antenatal glucocorticoid was associated with lower birthweight compared with exposure to 1–3 courses [46]. However, again in those retrospective studies treatments were non-randomly allocated. In contrast, a randomized prospective trial in 503 pregnant women found no association between repeated corticosteroid doses and birthweight or head circumference [44].

Antenatal Dexamethasone Therapy in Congenital Adrenal Hyperplasia

Maternal dexamethasone therapy effectively suppresses abnormal adrenal androgen production and virilization of the female fetus affected by congenital adrenal hyperplasia (CAH) [47]. Oral dexamethasone (0.02 mg/kg/day in three divided doses) should be started by 6–8 weeks' gestation and, depending on the results of karyotyping and mutation analysis, treatment is discontinued around 10 weeks' gestation in pregnancies with a male fetus, and around 14 weeks with an unaffected female fetus. Follow-up of the now over 1,000 treated infants may help identify any side effects of early and long-term antenatal glucocorticoid exposure [48–50]. Significant maternal side-effects are noted, including striae, acne, hirsutism, excessive weight gain, and mood fluctuations. However, there appears to be little adverse effect on the fetus. While occasional cases of intrauterine growth retardation have been reported, average birthweight, length and head circumference are normal in all studies. One study even reported larger birthlengths in treated offspring [50].

In rat studies, antenatal dexamethasone therapy also produced more aggressive postnatal behavior in the offspring [35]. However, in humans, a recent report found no significant effects of antenatal dexamethasone on detailed developmental outcomes [51]. An important difference may be that the majority of animal studies use doses that are one or two orders of magnitude above the doses recommended to treat pregnancies at risk for CAH [52].

In summary, currently it appears that only the highest, repeated antenatal steroid doses may have deleterious effects on human fetal growth. This does not exclude the possibility of long-term effects of lower steroid doses on metabolic disease risk. Prospective follow-up studies of subjects exposed to antenatal glucocorticoid therapy are in progress to detect any effects on blood pressure, body composition, insulin sensitivity and glucocorticoid secretion. Identification of effects of common genetic variations that regulate glucocorticoid secretion or activity, on antenatal growth rates and long-term outcomes could also provide important evidence for a common role of the glucocorticoid axis in the fetal origins of adult disease.

11β-Hydroxysteroid Dehydrogenase

A major source of interindividual variation in the effects of glucocorticoid exposure may arise from differences in activities of the 11β-hydroxysteroid dehydrogenase (11β-HSD) enzymes type 1 and 2, which shuttle active cortisol to inactive cortisone and vice versa [34]. In the fetus, placental β-HSD2 activity largely prevents any maternal cortisol crossing the placenta. Dexamethasone, a synthetic fluorinated steroid, is a poor substrate for 11β-HSD2, and the fetal effects of maternal dexamethasone therapy are therefore unlikely to vary with 11β-HSD2 activity. However, by controlling the effects of endogenous cortisol secretion on fetal growth and postnatal body fat and blood pressure, variations in placental and postnatal 11β-HSD activities could link low birthweight to adult hypertension and metabolic syndrome risk.

In rats, inhibition of placental 11β-HSD2 by giving the mother carbenoxelone exposes the fetus to excess glucocorticoids, and results in both a 20% reduction in birthweight and also higher mean arterial blood pressure in the adult offspring [53]. In humans, reduced placental 11β-HSD2 function is associated with pregnancy induced hypertension in the mother and low birthweight. Rare deleterious human mutations in placental 11β-HSD2 activity expose the fetus to excess maternal glucocorticoids and result in severely reduced fetal growth [54]. In a study of normal birthweight term infants, lower placental 11β-HSD2 activity was associated with lower offspring birthweight [55]. Another study in small preterm infants also reported a remarkably strong correlation between placental 11β-HSD2 activity and birthweight [56]. In that study, lower 11β-HSD2 activity was also associated with increased umbilical artery resistance, and it is possible that lower enzyme activity might represent a stress response to other causes of fetal growth restraint [57]. Associations between common functional variants in the 11β-HSD1 or 11β-HSD2 genes [58] could further demonstrate the importance of 11β-HSD activity to the links between fetal growth and long-term disease risks.

Programming of Adrenal Androgen Production

The adrenal androgens, dehydroepiandrosterone (DHEA) and DHEA-sulfate (DHEAS), are produced by the adrenal zona reticularis [59], and circulating DHEAS levels provide a convenient marker of rate of adrenal androgen production [60]. In parallel with adrenal glucocorticoid secretion, DHEAS production in low-birthweight subjects appears to follow a similar pattern from initial deficiency in the first few days of life to subsequent hypersecretion during later childhood. The consequences of ongoing adrenal androgen hypersecretion include potential effects on rate of maturation and puberty, and long-term risks for the polycystic ovary syndrome (PCOS) and insulin resistance.

Low DHEAS Levels in the Low-Birthweight Newborn

The adrenal cortex fetal zone is morphologically equivalent to the zona reticularis in older children and adults. The fetal zone does not express 3β-HSD (required for cortisol production), but does express P450scc and P450c17 (required to produce DHEAS). This fetal zone rapidly disappears during the first few weeks after birth and DHEA and DHEAS levels are usually undetectable [61, 62]. Adrenal androgen secretion rises again from around the age of 6 years onwards at 'adrenarche' [62].

Low-birthweight infants have relative hypoplasia of the fetal zone [63], and lower DHEAS levels in both plasma and urine during the first 24 h of life compared with normal birthweight infants [64, 65]. Norman et al. [66] studied 22 twin pregnancies, each with one IUGR twin and one normal birthweight twin. In each pair, the IUGR twin had lower DHEAS levels in umbilical arterial blood at birth than their larger twin, but cortisol levels were no different.

High DHEAS Levels following Low Birthweight

In contrast to the low DHEAS levels at birth, DHEAS levels are higher than average in older low-birthweight children. These findings have been consistently seen in case-control studies comparing small for gestational age (SGA) to normal birthweight children, in populations from: Sweden [67], Spain [68], Italy [69], and Finland [25]. Furthermore, in 8-year-old Belgian twins discordant for birthweight, the lower birthweight twin had on average 2-fold higher DHEAS levels than the larger birthweight twin [70]. In adults, higher DHEAS levels have been reported to correlate with higher fasting insulin levels in low-birthweight women, but not in men [23]. One large study showed no difference in DHEAS levels between short SGA children and control children with normal birthweight and normal stature [71]; in that study the effect of low birthweight on DHEAS levels could have been balanced by the larger current body size of the controls [72].

A recent large birth cohort study of unselected UK subjects (ALSPAC) described that higher DHEAS levels were not confined to the smallest birthweight infants, but rather there was a continuous inverse relationship between birthweight and DHEAS levels throughout the range of birthweights [26], i.e. similar to the relationships between birthweight and adult disease risks [3]. Together, the findings from both case control and population studies indicate that increased adrenal androgen secretion during childhood may be programmed by the combination of reduced fetal growth and rapid early postnatal weight gain.

The reason for this reversal in DHEAS levels in low-birthweight subjects, from low levels in the newborn to high levels in later childhood following adrenarche, is unknown. It has been suggested that the rise in adrenal androgen production during childhood follows an exponential curve and that its timing and amplitude might be set in early childhood [73]. Those conclusions were based on observations in girls with precocious puberty on LHRH-agonist treatment, and may therefore not be fully representative of normal children. Alternatively DHEAS levels could be regulated by weight gain, as the reversal in its levels appears to follow the typical pattern of rapid early postnatal weight gain that is seen in the majority of low-birthweight children.

Low birthweight, particularly if due to in utero growth restraint, is usually followed by a compensatory period of rapid, or 'catch-up', weight gain during early postnatal life [74]. In particular, it is this rapid weight gain during the first 3 years of life, and subsequent larger childhood size and adiposity [75], which appears to influence the onset of adrenarche (fig. 1). In the ALSPAC birth cohort, low birthweight followed by rapid early postnatal weight gain also led to higher insulin-like growth factor-I (IGF-I) levels at age 5 years [76], and lower insulin sensitivity at age 8 years [77]. IGF-I and insulin levels are higher in children with premature adrenarche than in control children [78–80], and could therefore link the combination of low birthweight and rapid infancy weight gain to the development of higher adrenal androgen production in later life activity [81].

Clinical Implications of Raised DHEAS Levels

Adrenarche is normally associated with the onset of mild clinical features of acne, pubic hair (pubarche) and body odor. In addition to these features, adrenarche has been observed to coincide with a mild growth acceleration, 'the mid-childhood growth spurt', between ages 6 and 8 years [82]. High levels of adrenal androgens, as occur in poorly controlled congenital adrenal hyperplasia (CAH), may trigger the activation of puberty. Programming of higher adrenal

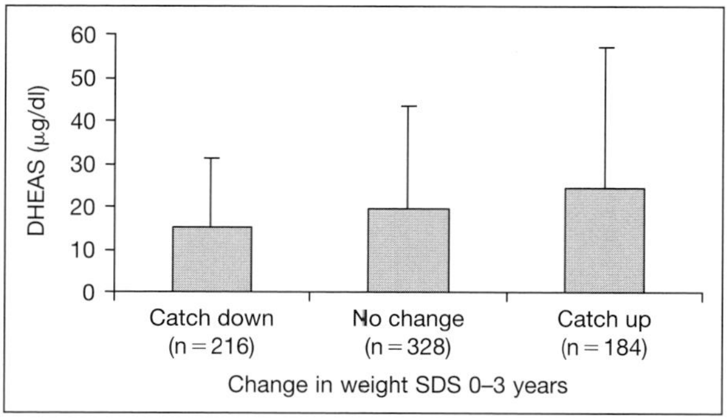

Fig. 1. Rapid weight gain between birth to 3 years predicts higher DHEAS levels at age 8 years (p trend: adjusted for weight at 8 years, $p = 0.002$). Catch up = Gain in weight SDS 0–3 years $>+0.67$; no change = -0.67 to $+0.67$; catch down = <-0.67. Geometric means +1 SD range. Reproduced from Ong [26].

androgen levels could therefore explain the tendency to earlier onset of puberty associated with low birthweight and rapid early postnatal growth [83, 84]. However, in most cases mild elevations in adrenal androgen levels probably have negligible effects on the onset and progression of puberty [85].

Early or exaggerated adrenal androgen secretion may lead to more marked clinical features of adrenal hyperandrogenism, and these are associated with other adverse effects on body composition, insulin resistance, and also increased risk of future progression to ovarian hyperandrogenism in the early years post-menarche.

Premature Pubarche

Premature pubarche is defined as the onset of pubic hair at age <8 years in girls, and <9 years in boys. In the exclusion of other pathology, such as non-classical CAH, virilizing tumors, or Cushing's syndrome, the cause appears to be simply a premature and most often exaggerated rise in adrenal androgen secretion [86]. The incidence is much higher in girls than in boys (up to 10:1) [87], although some of this excess could be due to presentation bias. It is likely that there is a wide ethnic variation in frequency of precocious pubarche [88], and studies are often reported from Mediterranean and African-American populations [86, 89, 90].

Girls who presented with precocious pubarche have increased risk for developing ovarian hyperandrogenism and other features of PCOS during the early years post-menarche [91]. These features include excessive virilization (acne and hirsutism), menstrual irregularity, and chronic anovulation, which may result in infertility. These risks are particularly high in precocious pubarche girls with history of low birthweight [92], and they also have increased biochemical markers for long-term risks of cardiovascular disease and type 2 diabetes, including hyperinsulinemia, dyslipidemia, and an abnormal adipocytokine pattern [93, 94].

Etiology of Precocious Pubarche

Case control studies showed an increased prevalence of low birthweight in precocious pubarche girls [92]. In these precocious pubarche subjects, as in the above studies of low-birthweight subjects with higher DHEAS levels, postnatal catch-up growth is a consistent feature [85]. Although they are not necessarily overweight, whole body DXA scans show that precocious pubarche girls have greater fat mass and central fat, and relatively reduced lean body mass compared with control girls with similar levels of BMI [95]. Excess central adiposity might be a direct consequence of excess androgens [96], or alternatively it might reflect the hyperinsulinemia that is co-present in such girls. Indeed, in precocious pubarche, as in PCOS, there has been debate as to whether hyperandrogenism or hyperinsulinism are etiological, as both these features are present, and in females hyperandrogenism can lead to hyperinsulinism and vice versa.

Genetic association studies using common functional variants have helped to demonstrate etiological roles for both increased androgen activity and hyperinsulinemia in precocious pubarche and in the risk of progression to ovarian hyperandrogenism. Shorter androgen receptor gene CAG repeat number confers increased androgen receptor sensitivity in vitro [97, 98], and is associated with conditions of increased androgen activity [99, 100]. Shorter CAG repeat length ($\leq$20 repeats) was associated with precocious pubarche in girls, and was an independent determinant for progression to ovarian hyperandrogenism following menarche [101]. Recognized population variation in the frequency of shorter androgen receptor CAG repeat alleles [102] could therefore contribute to population differences in the frequency of premature pubarche [88].

Increased severity of precocious pubarche in girls, including lower birthweight and hyperinsulinemia, have also been associated with the common insulin gene variable number of tandem repeat (VNTR) class I alleles [103]. Therefore, genetic predispositions to both increased insulin and androgen activity have etiological roles. In both of those genetic association studies, low birthweight was a separate independent cofactor for precocious pubarche risk or severity. Low birthweight could exacerbate both hyperinsulinemia by inducing insulin resistance, and also hyperandrogenemia by programming higher adrenal androgen secretion.

Therapeutic Studies in Girls with PCOS after Precocious Pubarche

A recent series of randomized open label trials of insulin sensitization and androgen receptor blockade therapies have added much to our understanding of the pathogenesis of precocious pubarche and risk for progressing to PCOS following low birthweight. Use of the insulin sensitizer metformin (1,275 mg daily for 6 months) in 16-year-old non-obese girls with previous precocious pubarche and current ovarian hyperandrogenism markedly reduced circulating insulin levels, androgen levels and hirsutism score, improved lipid profiles [104], and also restored ovulation in 78% of subjects [105].

In a similar population, monotherapy with low-dose flutamide (250 mg daily for 18 months) had no effect on insulin levels or menstrual irregularity, but improved lipid profiles and clinical features of hyperandrogenemia [106]. Of note, both androgen receptor blockade therapy and genetically reduced androgen receptor sensitivity [101] are associated with lower (rather than higher) circulating androgen levels. This physiologically unusual state (lower hormone levels in the presence of lower hormone receptor sensitivity) could be explained by a positive feedback effect of testosterone in promoting greater ovarian androgen secretion.

The marked additive effects of combined metformin and low dose flutamide (125 mg daily) therapies underline the separate contributions of both increased insulin and androgen activity in the pathogenesis of ovarian androgen excess (fig. 2) [107, 108]. In combined therapies, monthly ovulation rates increased within 9 months from below 10% to above 90%. Similar improvements were seen with the further addition of oral contraception, which is important as flutamide is contraindicated in pregnancy [109]. Finally, the rapid reversal of all the improvements in hormonal, biochemical and body compositional parameters on discontinuation of combined therapy (fig. 2) [108] indicates the continuing presence of a further yet unidentified underlying abnormality, and in particular a propensity to central fat accumulation that may be related to low birthweight, postnatal catch-up growth, genetic factors or their interactions.

Early Preventive Strategies

The relatively early clinical presentation of precocious pubarche in girls, together with available accurate characterization of the risk of progressing to more severe features of ovarian hyperandrogenism, allows the prediction and targeting of potential early interventions. Ibanez et al. recently reported a novel randomized open-label study of metformin (850 mg daily) treatment in 24 non-obese precocious pubarche girls with hyperinsulinemia and subclinical ovarian hyperandrogenism, starting early post-menarche (mean age 12.4 years), in order to

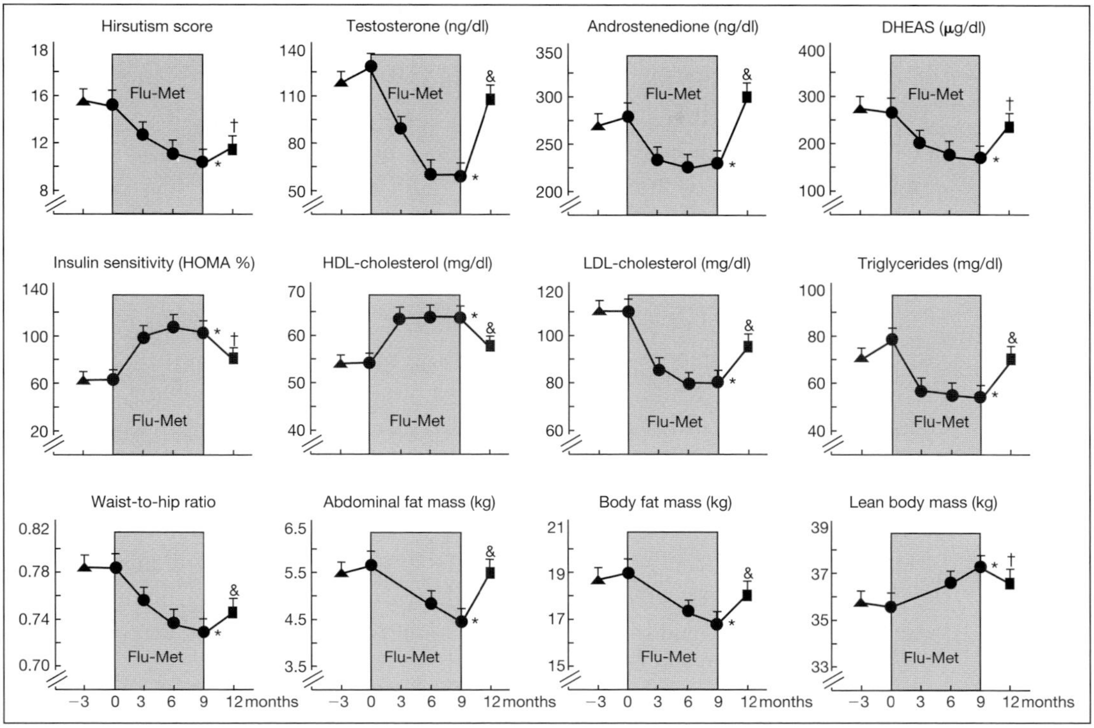

Fig. 2. Widespread beneficial effects of 9 months combined flutamide-metformin (Flu-Met) treatment in precocious pubarche girls with ovarian hyperandrogenism (n = 30; mean age 15.8 years), and subsequent deterioration on discontinuation (n = 16). *$p < 0.0001$ vs. 0 months (n = 30); †$p < 0.01$ vs. 9 months; or & $p < 0.001$ vs. 9 months (n = 16). None of the −3 vs. 0 month differences reached statistical significance (n = 14). Reproduced from Ibanez et al. [108].

prevent progression to overt PCOS [110]. These precocious pubarche girls were selected for low birthweight (<2.4 kg at term), and therefore high risk of progression. Over the 12 month study, in untreated girls features of insulin resistance, hyperandrogenemia, dyslipidemia, excess truncal fat, and reduced lean body mass all continued to diverge further away from normal; conversely in metformin-treated girls all these abnormalities showed significant improvements. Such positive results have encouraged the study of even earlier treatment strategies, at or soon after the onset of precocious pubarche (mean age 8.0 years) with low-dose metformin (425 mg daily); after 6 months significant beneficial effects have been observed on adrenal androgen levels, lipid profiles, reduced total and abdominal fat mass, and increased lean body mass [94].

Conclusions

The apparent consequences of low birthweight on later increases in both adrenal cortisol and adrenal androgen production may impact not only pubertal development, but they may also contribute to the longer-term disease risks described by studies of the fetal origins of adult disease. Further studies are needed to identify the precise metabolic pathways that are affected by low birthweight, and in particular how these may be further exaggerated by rapid 'catch-up' weight gain during early postnatal life.

The development of early and safe treatments for precocious pubarche in girls, and in particular early preventative strategies against progression to PCOS, may provide treatment models for the prevention of other longer-term consequences of low birthweight on metabolic disease risk. It may be easier to develop such treatment strategies in low-birthweight subjects with overt clinical features, such as in precocious pubarche girls, where efficacy has clearly perceived benefits to the patient. Transferring these strategies to the prevention of long-term consequences of the fetal origins of adult disease will require the development of robust markers of future disease risks, possibly including genetic markers, and also indicators of treatment response that are based on a clear understanding of the mechanisms involved.

Acknowledgments

I thank Lourdes Ibanez, Francis de Zegher and David Dunger for sharing many valuable discussions and comments.

References

1 Karn MN, Penrose LS: Birth weight and gestation time in relation to maternal age, parity and infant survival. Ann Eugenics 1951;16:147–158.
2 Barker DJ: Fetal growth and adult disease. Br J Obstet Gynaecol 1992;99:275–276.
3 Hales CN, Barker DJ: The thrifty phenotype hypothesis. Br Med Bull 2001;60:5–20.
4 Editorial: An overstretched hypothesis? Editorial. Lancet 2001;357:405.
5 Brosnan PG: The hypothalamic pituitary axis in the fetus and newborn. Semin Perinatol 2001; 25:371–384.
6 Yeh TF, Lin YJ, Lin HC, Huang CC, Hsieh WS, Lin CH, Tsai CH: Outcomes at school age after postnatal dexamethasone therapy for lung disease of prematurity. N Engl J Med 2004;350: 1304–1313.
7 Reinisch JM, Simon NG, Karow WG, Gandelman R: Prenatal exposure to prednisone in humans and animals retards intrauterine growth. Science 1978;202:436–438.
8 Pratt L, Magness RR, Phernetton T, Hendricks SK, Abbott DH, Bird IM: Repeated use of betamethasone in rabbits: Effects of treatment variation on adrenal suppression, pulmonary maturation, and pregnancy outcome. Am J Obstet Gynecol 1999;180:995–1005.

9 Jobe AH, Wada N, Berry LM, Ikegami M, Ervin MG: Single and repetitive maternal glucocorticoid exposures reduce fetal growth in sheep. Am J Obstet Gynecol 1998;178:880–885.
10 Eskola V, Lenko HL, Tammela O: Impaired adrenocortical function in very low birth weight infants after multiple pregnancies. Eur J Endocrinol 2003;149:529–534.
11 Ng PC, Lee CH, Lam CW, Ma KC, Fok TF, Chan IH, Wong E: Transient adrenocortical insufficiency of prematurity and systemic hypotension in very low birthweight infants. Arch Dis Child Fetal Neonatal Ed 2004;89:F119–F126.
12 Korte C, Styne D, Merritt TA, Mayes D, Wertz A, Helbock HJ: Adrenocortical function in the very low birth weight infant: Improved testing sensitivity and association with neonatal outcome. J Pediatr 1996;128:257–263.
13 Watterberg KL, Scott SM, Backstrom C, Gifford KL, Cook KL: Links between early adrenal function and respiratory outcome in preterm infants: Airway inflammation and patent ductus arteriosus. Pediatrics 2000;105:320–324.
14 Kari MA, Raivio KO, Stenman UH, Voutilainen R: Serum cortisol, dehydroepiandrosterone sulfate, and steroid-binding globulins in preterm neonates: Effect of gestational age and dexamethasone therapy. Pediatr Res 1996;40:319–324.
15 Hingre RV, Gross SJ, Hingre KS, Mayes DM, Richman RA: Adrenal steroidogenesis in very low birth weight preterm infants. J Clin Endocrinol Metab 1994;78:266–270.
16 Ng PC, Lam CW, Lee CH, Ma KC, Fok TF, Chan IH, Wong E: Reference ranges and factors affecting the human corticotropin-releasing hormone test in preterm, very low birth weight infants. J Clin Endocrinol Metab 2002;87:4621–4628.
17 Ng PC, Lam CW, Lee CH, Wong GW, Fok TF, Wong E, Chan IH, Ma KC: Changes of leptin and metabolic hormones in preterm infants: A longitudinal study in early postnatal life. Clin Endocrinol (Oxf) 2001;54:673–680.
18 Klemcke HG, Lunstra DD, Brown-Borg HM, Borg KE, Christenson RK: Association between low birth weight and increased adrenocortical function in neonatal pigs. J Anim Sci 1993;71:1010–1018.
19 Poore KR, Fowden AL: The effect of birth weight on hypothalamo-pituitary-adrenal axis function in juvenile and adult pigs. J Physiol 2003;547:107–116.
20 Phillips DI, Barker DJ, Fall CH, Seckl JR, Whorwood CB, Wood PJ, Walker BR: Elevated plasma cortisol concentrations: A link between low birth weight and the insulin resistance syndrome? J Clin Endocrinol Metab 1998;83:757–760.
21 Phillips DI, Walker BR, Reynolds RM, Flanagan DE, Wood PJ, Osmond C, Barker DJ, Whorwood CB: Low birth weight predicts elevated plasma cortisol concentrations in adults from 3 populations. Hypertension 2000;35:1301–1306.
22 Levitt NS, Lambert EV, Woods D, Hales CN, Andrew R, Seckl JR: Impaired glucose tolerance and elevated blood pressure in low birth weight, nonobese, young South African adults: Early programming of cortisol axis. J Clin Endocrinol Metab 2000;85:4611–4618.
23 Szathmari M, Vasarhelyi B, Tulassay T: Effect of low birth weight on adrenal steroids and carbohydrate metabolism in early adulthood. Horm Res 2001;55:172–178.
24 Walker BR, Irving RJ, Andrew R, Belton NR: Contrasting effects of intrauterine growth retardation and premature delivery on adult cortisol secretion and metabolism in man. Clin Endocrinol (Oxf) 2002;57:351–355.
25 Tenhola S, Martikainen A, Rahiala E, Parviainen M, Halonen P, Voutilainen R: Increased adrenocortical and adrenomedullary hormonal activity in 12-year-old children born small for gestational age. J Pediatr 2002;141:477–482.
26 Ong KK, Potau N, Petry CJ, Jones R, Ness AR, Honour JW, de Zegher F, Ibanez L, Dunger DB: Opposing influences of prenatal and postnatal weight gain on adrenarche in normal boys and girls. J Clin Endocrinol Metab 2004;89:2647–2651.
27 Honour JW: Hypothalamic-pituitary-adrenal axis. Resp Med 1994;88(suppl A):9–15.
28 Jackson JA, Wailoo MP, Thompson JR, Petersen SA: Early physiological development of infants with intrauterine growth retardation. Arch Dis Child 2004;89:F46–F50.
29 Clark PM, Hindmarsh PC, Shiell AW, Law CM, Honour JW, Barker DJ: Size at birth and adrenocortical function in childhood. Clin Endocrinol (Oxf) 1996;45:721–726.

30 Fall CH, Dennison E, Cooper C, Pringle J, Kellingray SD, Hindmarsh P: Does birth weight predict adult serum cortisol concentrations? Twenty-four-hour profiles in the United kingdom 1920–1930 Hertfordshire Birth Cohort. J Clin Endocrinol Metab 2002;87:2001–2007.
31 Reynolds RM, Walker BR, Syddall HE, Andrew R, Wood PJ, Whorwood CB, Phillips DI: Altered control of cortisol secretion in adult men with low birth weight and cardiovascular risk factors. J Clin Endocrinol Metab 2001;86:245–250.
32 Kajantie E, Eriksson J, Barker DJ, Forsen T, Osmond C, Wood PJ, Andersson S, Dunkel L, Phillips DI: Birth size, gestational age and adrenal function in adult life: Studies of dexamethasone suppression and ACTH1–24 stimulation. Eur J Endocrinol 2003;149:569–575.
33 Levitt NS, Lindsay RS, Holmes MC, Seckl JR: Dexamethasone in the last week of pregnancy attenuates hippocampal glucocorticoid receptor gene expression and elevates blood pressure in the adult offspring in the rat. Neuroendocrinology 1996;64:412–418.
34 Edwards CR, Benediktsson R, Lindsay RS, Seckl JR: 11 beta-Hydroxysteroid dehydrogenases: Key enzymes in determining tissue-specific glucocorticoid effects. Steroids 1996;61: 263–269.
35 Reinisch JM, Simon NG, Gandelman R: Prenatal exposure to prednisone permanently alters fighting behavior of female mice. Pharmacol Biochem Behav 1980;12:213–216.
36 Moritz KM, Johnson K, Douglas-Denton R, Wintour EM, Dodic M: Maternal glucocorticoid treatment programs alterations in the renin-angiotensin system of the ovine fetal kidney. Endocrinology 2002;143:4455–4463.
37 Hales CN, Barker DJ, Clark PM, Cox LJ, Fall C, Osmond C, Winter PD: Fetal and infant growth and impaired glucose tolerance at age 64. BMJ 1991;303:1019–1022.
38 Crowley P: Prophylactic corticosteroids for preterm birth (Cochrane review). Oxford, The Cochrane Library, 2001, Issue 3, Update Software.
39 NIH Consensus Development Panel: Effect of corticosteroids for fetal maturation on perinatal outcomes. JAMA 1995;273:413–418.
40 Smolders-de Haas H, Neuvel J, Schmand B, Treffers PE, Koppe JG, Hoeks J: Physical development and medical history of children who were treated antenatally with corticosteroids to prevent respiratory distress syndrome: A 10- to 12-year follow-up. Pediatrics 1990;86: 65–70.
41 Dessens AB, Haas HS, Koppe JG: Twenty-year follow-up of antenatal corticosteroid treatment. Pediatrics 2000;105:E77.
42 Doyle LW, Ford GW, Davis NM, Callanan C: Antenatal corticosteroid therapy and blood pressure at 14 years of age in preterm children. Clin Sci (Lond) 2000;98:137–142.
43 Doyle LW, Ford GW, Rickards AL, Kelly EA, Davis NM, Callanan C, Olinsky A: Antenatal corticosteroids and outcome at 14 years of age in children with birth weight less than 1501 grams. Pediatrics 2000;106:E2.
44 Guinn DA, Atkinson MW, Sullivan L, Lee M, MacGregor S, Parilla BV, Davies J, Hanlon-Lundberg K, Simpson L, Stone J, Wing D, Ogasawara K, Muraskas J: Single vs weekly courses of antenatal corticosteroids for women at risk of preterm delivery: A randomized controlled trial. JAMA 2001;286:1581–1587.
45 French NP, Hagan R, Evans SF, Godfrey M, Newnham JP: Repeated antenatal corticosteroids: size at birth and subsequent development. Am J Obstet Gynecol 1999;180:114–121.
46 Lam PM, Yuen PM, Lau TK, Leung TN: Relationship between birthweight and repeated courses of antenatal corticosteroids. Aust NZ J Obstet Gynaecol 2001;41:281–284.
47 David M, Forest MG: Prenatal treatment of congenital adrenal hyperplasia resulting from 21-hydroxylase deficiency. J Pediatr 1984;105:799–803.
48 New MI, Carlson A, Obeid J, Marshall I, Cabrera MS, Goseco A, Lin-Su K, Putnam AS, Wei JQ, Wilson RC: Prenatal diagnosis for congenital adrenal hyperplasia in 532 pregnancies. J Clin Endocrinol Metab 2001;86:5651–5657.
49 Forest MG, Morel Y, David M: Prenatal treatment of congenital adrenal hyperplasia. Trends Endocrinol Metab 1998;9:284–289.
50 Lajic S, Wedell A, Bui TH, Ritzen EM, Holst M: Long-term somatic follow-up of prenatally treated children with congenital adrenal hyperplasia. J Clin Endocrinol Metab 1998;83: 3872–3880.

51 Meyer-Bahlburg HF, Dolezal C, Baker SW, Carlson AD, Obeid JS, New MI: Cognitive and motor development of children with and without congenital adrenal hyperplasia after early-prenatal dexamethasone. J Clin Endocrinol Metab 2004;89:610–614.
52 Dodic M, Tersteeg M, Jefferies A, Wintour EM, Moritz K: Prolonged low-dose dexamethasone treatment, in early gestation, does not alter blood pressure or renal function in adult sheep. J Endocrinol 2003;179:275–280.
53 Lindsay RS, Lindsay RM, Edwards CR, Seckl JR: Inhibition of 11-beta-hydroxysteroid dehydrogenase in pregnant rats and the programming of blood pressure in the offspring. Hypertension 1996;27:1200–1204.
54 Edwards CR, Benediktsson R, Lindsay RS, Seckl JR: Dysfunction of placental glucocorticoid barrier: Link between fetal environment and adult hypertension? Lancet 1993;341:355–357.
55 Stewart PM, Rogerson FM, Mason JI: Type 2 11 beta-hydroxysteroid dehydrogenase messenger ribonucleic acid and activity in human placenta and fetal membranes: Its relationship to birth weight and putative role in fetal adrenal steroidogenesis. J Clin Endocrinol Metab 1995;80:885–890.
56 Kajantie E, Dunkel L, Turpeinen U, Stenman UH, Wood PJ, Nuutila M, Andersson S: Placental 11 beta-hydroxysteroid dehydrogenase-2 and fetal cortisol/cortisone shuttle in small preterm infants. J Clin Endocrinol Metab 2003;88:493–500.
57 Bertram C, Trowern AR, Copin N, Jackson AA, Whorwood CB: The maternal diet during pregnancy programs altered expression of the glucocorticoid receptor and type 2 11beta-hydroxysteroid dehydrogenase: Potential molecular mechanisms underlying the programming of hypertension in utero. Endocrinology 2001;142:2841–2853.
58 Gelernter-Yaniv L, Feng N, Sebring NG, Hochberg Z, Yanovski JA: Associations between a polymorphism in the 11 beta hydroxysteroid dehydrogenase type I gene and body composition. Int J Obes Relat Metab Disord 2003;27:983–986.
59 Endoh A, Kristiansen SB, Casson PR, Buster JE, Hornsby PJ: The zona reticularis is the site of biosynthesis of dehydroepiandrosterone and dehydroepiandrosterone sulfate in the adult human adrenal cortex resulting from its low expression of 3 beta-hydroxysteroid dehydrogenase. J Clin Endocrinol Metab 1996;81:3558–3565.
60 Meikle AW, Daynes RA, Araneo BA: Adrenal androgen secretion and biologic effects. Endocrinol.Metab.Clin.North.Am 1991;20:381–400.
61 Mesiano S, Jaffe RB: Developmental and functional biology of the primate fetal adrenal cortex. Endocr Rev 1997;18:378–403.
62 Babalola AA, Ellis G: Serum dehydroepiandrosterone sulfate in a normal pediatric population. Clin. Biochem 1985;18:184–189.
63 Naeye RL: Malnutrition: Probable cause of fetal growth retardation. Arch Pathol 1965;79:284–291.
64 Turnipseed MR, Bentley K, Reynolds JW: Serum dehydroepiandrosterone sulfate in premature infants and infants with intrauterine growth retardation. J Clin Endocrinol Metab 1976;43: 1219–1225.
65 Reynolds JW, Mirkin BL: Urinary steroid levels in newborn infants with intrauterine growth retardation. J Clin Endocrinol Metab 1973;36:576–581.
66 Norman RJ, Joubert SM: Fetal adrenal gland maturation in growth-retarded twin pregnancies. Acta Genet Med Gemellol (Roma) 1982;31:259–262.
67 Dahlgren J, Boguszewski M, Rosberg S, Albertsson-Wikland K: Adrenal steroid hormones in short children born small for gestational age. Clin Endocrinol (Oxf) 1998;49:353–361.
68 Ibanez L, Potau N, Marcos MV, de Zegher F: Exaggerated adrenarche and hyperinsulinism in adolescent girls born small for gestational age. J Clin Endocrinol Metab 1999;84:4739–4741.
69 Ghirri P, Bernardini M, Vuerich M, Cuttano AM, Coccoli L, Merusi I, Ciulli C, D'Accavio L, Bottone U, Boldrini A: Adrenarche, pubertal development, age at menarche and final height of full-term, born small for gestational age (SGA) girls. Gynecol Endocrinol 2001;15:91–97.
70 Francois I, de Zegher F: Adrenarche and fetal growth. Pediatr Res 1997;41:440–442.
71 Boonstra VH, Mulder PG, de Jong FH, Hokken-Koelega AC: Serum dehydroepiandrosterone sulfate levels and pubarche in short children born small for gestational age before and during growth hormone treatment. J Clin Endocrinol Metab 2004;89:712–717.
72 Jabbar M, Pugliese M, Fort P, Recker B, Lifshitz F: Excess weight and precocious pubarche in children: Alterations of the adrenocortical hormones. J Am Coll Nutr 1991;10:289–296.

73 Palmert MR, Hayden DL, Mansfield MJ, Crigler JF Jr, Crowley WF Jr, Chandler DW, Boepple PA: The longitudinal study of adrenal maturation during gonadal suppression: Evidence that adrenarche is a gradual process. J Clin Endocrinol Metab 2001;86:4536–4542.
74 Ong KK, Preece MA, Emmett PM, Ahmed ML, Dunger DB: Size at birth and early childhood growth in relation to maternal smoking, parity and infant breast-feeding: Longitudinal birth cohort study and analysis. Pediatr Res 2002;52:863–867.
75 Ong KK, Ahmed ML, Emmett PM, Preece MA, Dunger DB, the ALSPAC Study Team: Association between postnatal catch-up growth and obesity in childhood: Prospective cohort study. BMJ 2000;320:967–971.
76 Ong KK, Kratzsch J, Kiess W, the-ALSPAC-Study-Team, Dunger DB: Circulating IGF-I levels in childhood are related to both current body composition and early postnatal growth rate. J Clin Endocrinol Metab 2002;87:1041–1044.
77 Ong KK, Petry CJ, Emmett PM, Sandhu MS, Kiess W, Hales CN, Ness AR, the ALSPAC Study Team, Dunger DB: Insulin sensitivity and secretion in normal children related to size at birth, postnatal growth, and plasma insulin-like growth factor-I levels. Diabetologia 2004;47: 1064–1070.
78 Ibanez L, Potau N, Zampolli M, Rique S, Saenger P, Carrascosa A: Hyperinsulinemia and decreased insulin-like growth factor-binding protein-1 are common features in prepubertal and pubertal girls with a history of premature pubarche. J Clin Endocrinol Metab 1997;82:2283–2288.
79 Silfen ME, Manibo AM, Ferin M, McMahon DJ, Levine LS, Oberfield SE: Elevated free IGF-I levels in prepubertal Hispanic girls with premature adrenarche: Relationship with hyperandrogenism and insulin sensitivity. J Clin Endocrinol Metab 2002;87:398–403.
80 Denburg MR, Silfen ME, Manibo AM, Chin D, Levine LS, Ferin M, McMahon DJ, Go C, Oberfield SE: Insulin sensitivity and the insulin-like growth factor system in prepubertal boys with premature adrenarche. J Clin Endocrinol Metab 2002;87:5604–5609.
81 Zhang LH, Rodriguez H, Ohno S, Miller WL: Serine phosphorylation of human P450c17 increases 17,20-lyase activity: Implications for adrenarche and the polycystic ovary syndrome. Proc Natl Acad Sci USA 1995;92:10619–10623.
82 Tanner JM, Cameron N: Investigation of the mid-growth spurt in height, weight and limb circumferences in single-year velocity data from the London, 1966–1967 growth survey. Ann Hum Biol 1980;7:565–577.
83 Adair LS: Size at birth predicts age at menarche. Pediatrics 2001;107:e59.
84 Mills JL, Shiono PH, Shapiro LR, Crawford PB, Rhoads GG: Early growth predicts timing of puberty in boys: Results of a 14-year nutrition and growth study. J Pediatr 1986;109:543–547.
85 Ibanez L, Virdis R, Potau N, Zampolli M, Ghizzoni L, Albisu MA, Carrascosa A, Bernasconi S, Vicens Calvet E: Natural history of premature pubarche: An auxological study. J Clin Endocrinol Metab 1992;74:254–257.
86 Ibanez L, Dimartino-Nardi J, Potau N, Saenger P: Premature adrenarche – Normal variant or forerunner of adult disease? Endocr Rev 2000;21:671–696.
87 Sigurjonsdottir TJ, Hayles AB: Premature pubarche. Clin Pediatr (Philad) 1968;7:29–33.
88 Herman Giddens ME, Slora EJ, Wasserman RC, Bourdony CJ, Bhapkar MV, Koch GG, Hasemeier CM: Secondary sexual characteristics and menses in young girls seen in office practice: A study from the Pediatric Research in Office Settings network. Pediatrics 1997;99:505–512.
89 DiMartino-Nardi J: Pre- and postpuberal findings in premature adrenarche. J Pediatr Endocrinol Metab 2000;13(suppl 5):1265–1269.
90 Dacou-Voutetakis C, Dracopoulou M: High incidence of molecular defects of the CYP21 gene in patients with premature adrenarche. J Clin Endocrinol Metab 1999;84:1570–1574.
91 Ibanez L, Potau N, Virdis R, Zampolli M, Terzi C, Gussinye M, Carrascosa A, Vicens Calvet E: Postpubertal outcome in girls diagnosed of premature pubarche during childhood: Increased frequency of functional ovarian hyperandrogenism. J Clin Endocrinol Metab 1993;76:1599–1603.
92 Ibanez L, Potau N, Francois I, de Zegher F: Precocious pubarche, hyperinsulinism, and ovarian hyperandrogenism in girls: Relation to reduced fetal growth. J Clin Endocrinol Metab 1998;83: 3558–3562.
93 Ibanez L, Potau N, Chacon P, Pascual C, Carrascosa A: Hyperinsulinaemia, dyslipaemia and cardiovascular risk in girls with a history of premature pubarche. Diabetologia 1998;41:1057–1063.

94 Ibanez L, Valls C, Marcos MV, Ong KK, Dunger DB, de Zegher F: Insulin Sensitization for girls with precocious pubarche and with risk for polycystic ovary syndrome: Effects of prepubertal initiation and postpubertal discontinuation of metformin. J Clin Endocrinol Metab 2004;89:4331–4337.
95 Ibanez L, Ong K, de Zegher F, Marcos MV, del Rio L, Dunger DB: Fat distribution in non-obese girls with and without precocious pubarche: Central adiposity related to insulinaemia and androgenaemia from prepuberty to postmenarche. Clin Endocrinol (Oxf) 2003;58:372–379.
96 Elbers JM, Asscheman H, Seidell JC, Megens JA, Gooren LJ: Long-term testosterone administration increases visceral fat in female to male transsexuals. J Clin Endocrinol Metab 1997;82: 2044–2047.
97 Chamberlain NL, Driver ED, Miesfeld RL: The length and location of CAG trinucleotide repeats in the androgen receptor N-terminal domain affect transactivation function. Nucl Acids Res 1994;22:3181–3186.
98 Choong CS, Kemppainen JA, Zhou ZX, Wilson EM: Reduced androgen receptor gene expression with first exon CAG repeat expansion. Mol Endocrinol 1996;10:1527–1535.
99 Hickey T, Chandy A, Norman RJ: The androgen receptor CAG repeat polymorphism and X-chromosome inactivation in Australian Caucasian women with infertility related to polycystic ovary syndrome. J Clin Endocrinol Metab 2002;87:161–165.
100 Dejager S, Bry-Gauillard H, Bruckert E, Eymard B, Salachas F, LeGuern E, Tardieu S, Chadarevian R, Giral P, Turpin G: A comprehensive endocrine description of Kennedy's disease revealing androgen insensitivity linked to CAG repeat length. J Clin Endocrinol Metab 2002;87:3893–3901.
101 Ibanez L, Ong KK, Mongan N, Jaaskelainen J, Marcos MV, Hughes IA, De Zegher F, Dunger DB: Androgen receptor gene CAG repeat polymorphism in the development of ovarian hyperandrogenism. J Clin Endocrinol Metab 2003;88:3333–3338.
102 Edwards A, Hammond HA, Jin L, Caskey CT, Chakraborty R: Genetic variation at five trimeric and tetrameric tandem repeat loci in four human population groups. Genomics 1992;12:241–253.
103 Ibanez L, Ong K, Potau N, Marcos MV, de Zegher F, Dunger D: Insulin gene variable number of tandem repeat genotype and the low birth weight, precocious pubarche, and hyperinsulinism sequence. J Clin Endocrinol Metab 2001;86:5788–5793.
104 Ibanez L, Valls C, Potau N, Marcos MV, de Zegher F: Sensitisation to insulin in adolescent girls to normalize hirsutism, hyperandrogenism, oligomenorrhea, dyslipidemia and hyperinsulinaemia after precocious pubarche. J Clin Endocrinol Metab 2000;85:3526–3530.
105 Ibanez L, Valls C, Ferrer A, Marcos MV, Rodriguez-Hierro F, de Zegher F: Sensitization to insulin induces ovulation in nonobese adolescents with anovulatory hyperandrogenism. J Clin Endocrinol Metab 2001;86:3595–3598.
106 Ibanez L, Potau N, Marcos MV, de Zegher F: Treatment of hirsutism, hyperandrogenism, oligomenorrhea, dyslipidemia, and hyperinsulinism in nonobese, adolescent girls: Effect of flutamide. J Clin Endocrinol Metab 2000;85:3251–3255.
107 Ibanez L, Valls C, Ferrer A, Ong K, Dunger DB, De Zegher F: Additive effects of insulin-sensitizing and anti-androgen treatment in young, nonobese women with hyperinsulinism, hyperandrogenism, dyslipidemia, and anovulation. J Clin Endocrinol Metab 2002;87:2870–2874.
108 Ibanez L, Ong KK, Ferrer A, Amin R, Dunger DB, de Zegher F: Low-dose flutamide-metformin therapy reverses insulin resistance and reduces fat mass in nonobese adolescents with ovarian hyperandrogenism. J Clin Endocrinol Metab 2003;88:2600–2606.
109 Ibanez L, de Zegher F: Ethinylestradiol-drospirenone, flutamide-metformin, or both for adolescents and women with hyperinsulinemic hyperandrogenism: Opposite effects on adipocytokines and body adiposity. J Clin Endocrinol Metab 2004;89:1592–1597.
110 Ibanez L, Ferrer A, Ong K, Amin R, Dunger D, de Zegher F: Insulin sensitization early after menarche prevents progression from precocious pubarche to polycystic ovary syndrome. J Pediatr 2004;144:23–29.

Dr. Ken K. Ong
Department of Paediatrics, University of Cambridge, Addenbrooke's Hospital
Level 8, Box 116, Cambridge CB2 2QQ (UK)
Tel. +44 0 1223 763405, Fax +44 0 1223 336996, E-Mail ko224@cam.ac.uk

Delemarre-van de Waal HA (ed): Abnormalities in Puberty. Scientific and Clinical Advances.
Endocr Dev. Basel, Karger, 2005, vol 8, pp 54–66

Puberty and Fertility in Congenital Adrenal Hyperplasia

B.J. Otten[a], *M.M.L. Stikkelbroeck*[b], *H.L. Claahsen-van der Grinten*[a], *A.R.M.M. Hermus*[b]

Departments of [a]Pediatric Endocrinology, and [b]Endocrinology, University Hospital St. Radboud, Nijmegen, The Netherlands

Abstract

Congenital adrenal hyperplasia (CAH) is a disorder of adrenal steroid synthesis. The symptoms and signs of CAH depend on the degree of enzyme deficiency; severe salt-wasting (SW) form, less severe simple virilizing (SV) form and mild nonclassic (NC) form. In this paper, puberty and fertility in CAH are discussed. The time of onset of puberty and progress of pubertal development is quite normal, except in NC patients (earlier). Also the age of menarche in CAH girls is normal, but it can depend on the level of therapeutic control. In prepuberty, bone age is advanced. In puberty, peak height velocity is normal but occurs at a younger age and can therefore be considered to be low (compared to healthy early maturers). In puberty there seems to be an increased sensitivity for glucocorticoids leading to growth inhibition. All three above factors can play a role in reducing adult height. Subfertility is frequently found in both female and male CAH patients. In females, the pregnancy rate depends on the severity of 21-hydroxylase deficiency (SW<SV<NC). Adrenal progestagens and androgens are the main cause of disturbed ovarian activity. In addition psychosexual problems (e.g. as a result of genital surgery) are an important factor. In males, the main cause of subfertiltiy is the presence of testicular adrenal rest tumors, which are thought to originate from aberrant adrenal tissue and respond to treatment with glucocorticoids. Although in general fertility is not a paediatric item, in CAH most fertility problems have their origins in childhood years. Therefore prevention of subfertility has to be implemented as a treatment goal in paediatric endocrinology from the start of puberty.

Congenital adrenal hyperplasia (CAH) is a disorder of adrenal steroid synthesis. In 95% of the cases, it is caused by 21-hydroxylase deficiency. This type of enzymatic deficiency leads to cortisol deficiency and (in most cases)

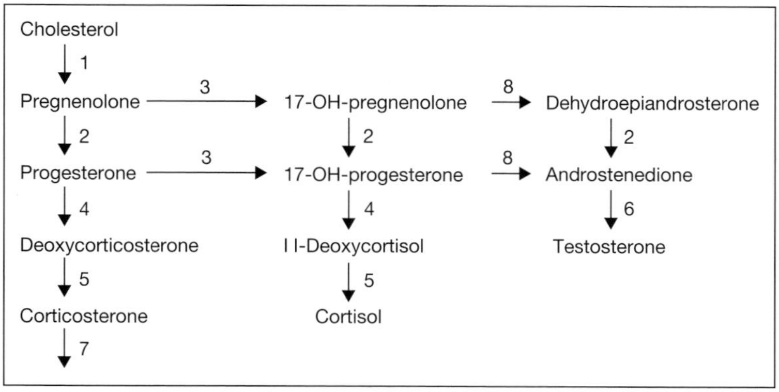

Fig. 1. Simplified scheme of adrenal steroidogenesis: (1) (cholesterol) side chain cleavage enzyme/steroidogenic autoregulatory protein (StAR); (2) 3β-hydroxysteroid-dehydrogenase; (3) 17-hydroxylase; (4) 21-hydroxylase; (5) 11-hydroxylase; (6) 17β-hydroxysteroid-dehydrogenase; (7) 18-dehydrogenase; (8) 17,20-lyase. Deficiency of the StAR protein or one of the enzymes 2–5 leads to congenital adrenal hyperplasia (CAH); 21-hydroxylase deficiency accounts for 95% of all CAH cases.

aldosterone deficiency. The compensatory increase in ACTH secretion by the pituitary gland leads to stimulation of the adrenals and, consequently, overproduction of androgens [1]. Figure 1 gives an overview of adrenal steroid synthesis.

The symptoms and signs of CAH depend on the degree of enzyme deficiency. For 21-hydroxylase deficiency, this results in a broad clinical picture: complete 21-hydroxylase deficiency leads to absence of cortisol and aldosterone, and salt-wasting crisis in the newborn period. The androgen excess results in prenatal virilization of the external genitalia in females (classic salt-wasting form: SW). Less severe 21-hydroxylase deficiency results in milder cortisol deficiency and milder prenatal androgen excess, with prenatal virilization in females, but no aldosterone deficiency (classic simple virilizing form: SV). Patients with the mildest forms present with symptoms caused by androgen excess only: pseudoprecocious puberty, hirsutism, menstrual irregularities and infertility, all of which are most readily detected in women (non-classic form) [1].

In this paper puberty and fertility in CAH are discussed.

Time of Onset of Puberty and Progress of Pubertal Development

In patients with classic CAH, the time of onset of puberty, defined as a testicular volume ≥4 ml in males and a Tanner breast stage 2 in females [2], is quite normal: for boys the mean age is around 11 years and for girls around 10 years [3–5], which is in the normal range. In patients with non-classic CAH the time of onset of puberty is reported to be somewhat earlier [3]. The mean duration of puberty is reported to be normal [3, 5].

In most studies in CAH girls, a normal mean age of menarche is reported [6–12], but these data may be misleading because by definition only the patients who did experience menarche were included. In CAH women, delayed menarche can be associated with poor therapeutic control: two reports compared age at menarche between adequately and poorly controlled patients and showed that in the latter, the mean age at menarche was higher [6, 9]. Although these differences were not statistically significant, likely as a result of the small numbers, they suggest that therapeutic control might affect the age of menarche.

Growth

Growth and Bone Maturation before Puberty

The mean height of CAH patients in late pre-puberty (7–10 years) is generally similar to the population mean except for nonclassic males who are somewhat taller [4, 13]. During the whole prepubertal period, bone age is advanced in both male and female SV and SW patients, probably as a result of androgen exposure. The ratio of bone age vs. chronological age (BA/CA ratio) is maximal at the age of 8 years in SW patients (1.39 for boys, 1.29 for girls) [13]. In SV patients, bone age is even more advanced (BA/CA ratio 2.17 for boys at 4 years, 1.5 for girls at age 7 years) [13]. The difference between SV and SW can be explained by the fact that SV patients (especially boys) are usually diagnosed only after they have been exposed to androgen excess during several years.

Consequently, bone age advancement at the onset of puberty (present in all CAH patients) is most pronounced in male SV patients [13]. This bone age advancement already prior to puberty results in a diminished adult height expectancy.

Growth during Puberty

Pubertal growth patterns in CAH have been described in detail by Hargitai et al. [13]. They analyzed childhood and pubertal growth in 341 patients with classic CAH. They showed that peak height velocity (PHV) in CAH boys and girls was normal, but that it occurred at an earlier age compared with the normal population. Since early maturing children usually reach a higher PHV compared with normal maturers [2], the PHV in CAH can be considered to be low compared to healthy early maturers [13]. This early occurring relatively low PHV may result in a reduction of final height.

Adult Height

Predicted adult height at onset of puberty is reported as being below the population mean with a variation between −0.5 and −1.5 SD [3, 4]. Adult height in CAH is reduced in comparison to reference and individual target height: Eugster et al. [14], in a meta-analysis, found a reduction of 1.37 SD in classic CAH. In some studies [3, 4] a lower adult height in boys (−1.3 SD) than in girls (−0.9 SD) is reported, with SV males having the lowest adult heights. This may be due to the late diagnosis leading to most pronounced advancement in bone age.

Susceptibility to Glucocorticoids

Another important item with respect to the attainment of adult height is the sensitivity of growth for glucocorticoid therapy. Previous studies have shown a negative correlation between glucocorticoid dose and growth velocity in the first year(s) of life [15, 16]. With respect to (pre-)puberty, Stikkelbroeck et al. [17] demonstrated that the negative effects of glucocorticoid medication were also marked between 8 and 14 years. So, while in the early prepubertal years (<8 years) undertreatment with an advancement of bone age has to be avoided, in the years before the onset of puberty and during puberty there is a greater risk for overtreatment with negative consequences for adult height expectations.

Precocious Puberty

While CAH is a recognized cause of pseudo precocious puberty, in some patients with CAH exposure to adrenal androgens may lead to early maturation of the hypothalamic-pituitary-gonadal axis and central precocious puberty. The diagnosis of central precocious puberty can be made on the basis of testicular enlargement in the boys and breast development in the girls. Gonadotropin levels are in the normal pubertal range, both basally and in response to GnRH stimulation. In these cases treatment with GnRH analogues is effective in arresting central puberty [18, 19]. With GnRH analogues treatment testis size decreased in the males, and breast development regressed in the females with a significant decrease in linear growth rate and rate of bone maturation and ultimately an increase in predicted adult height [18, 19]. However, during this treatment an extreme deceleration of growth rate may occur. A possible option for counteracting this effect may be addition of growth hormone (GH) to the therapy. Quintos et al. [20] compared the results of GH treatment in addition to GnRH analogue therapy in 8 pubertal CAH patients with matched controls and found a persistent increase of growth velocity over 2 years treatment and an increase of predicted adult height (PAH) from 159 to 170 cm. These results, however, have to be confirmed in larger studies. Until then GH treatment is far from being a standard therapy in the management of patients with CAH.

Fertility in Females

In women with CAH due to 21-hydroxylase deficiency, fertility seems to be reduced, based on reports of menstrual disorders, decreased pregnancy rates and decreased live-birth rates. Most reports about pregnancies in female patients with classic 21-hydroxylase deficiency are case reports, only a few reports provide pregnancy rates or live birth rates in large populations of CAH patients [6–8, 21–24]: the live-birth rate in classic SW CAH patients is 0–10%, in SV patients 33–50%, and in non-classic patients 63–90%. In the general population or in age-matched controls, pregnancy rates or live-birth rates are 65–91% [6, 7, 22, 23]. Data on fertility in patients with non-classic 21-hydroxylase deficiency may be biased by the fact that they are predominantly derived from studies in patients in whom the diagnosis of CAH was made after referral for subfertility and/or symptoms of hyperandrogenism. In the paper of Feldman et al. [25] reporting on 53 non-classic patients, 10 of the 20 patients who desired pregnancy already conceived before the diagnosis was made, whereas the rest did after initiation of hydrocortisone therapy (1 patient required also clomiphene citrate). Also, Birnbaum and Rose [26], reporting on 48 non-classic patients who presented with irregular menses and/or subfertility, found that the pregnancy rate was 93% (corrected for additional problems compromising fertility) after prednisone therapy (and in some cases additional clomiphene citrate).

Causes of Impaired Fertility in Women with CAH Due to 21-Hydroxylase Deficiency

Several factors have been suggested to contribute to impaired fertility in CAH females: adrenal overproduction of androgens and progestins (17-hydroxyprogesterone and progesterone), ovarian hyperandrogenism, polycystic ovary syndrome, ovarian adrenal rest tumors, genital surgery, and psychological factors such as delayed psychosexual development, reduced sexual activity and low maternal feelings.

Androgen overproduction by the adrenal gland can affect ovarian activity by inducing hypogonadotropism. However, unlike in CAH men [27–30], in CAH women hypogonadotropism has only rarely been reported.

The hypothesis that androgen excess has a negative (direct and/or indirect) effect on ovulation is supported by the finding that suppression of adrenal

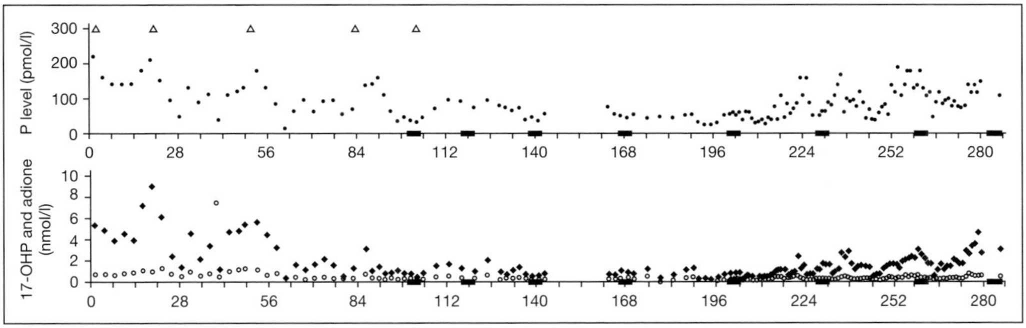

Fig. 2. Salivary levels of progesterone (P, black dots), 17 OH-progesterone (17-OHP, black diamonds) and androstenedione (adione, open circles) in a 15.5-year-old female patient with classic salt-wasting 21-hydroxylase deficiency and amenorrhea. Menstrual bleeding is indicated as black bars. At the start of the sampling, morning salivary levels of 17-OHP and P were increased and levels of androstenedione were in the normal range. To optimize adrenal suppression, hydrocortisone dose was gradually increased from 10.0 to 18.0 mg/m^2 in increments of 2 mg/m^2 (3 mg) per month (open triangles). Next, the evening hydrocortisone dose was replaced by dexamethasone. After 3 months, salivary levels of 17-OHP and P were in the normal range for healthy females or mildly elevated and the first vaginal bleeding occurred. Four months after menarche, a biphasic pattern in progesterone levels was found, suggesting ovulatory cycle. According to Stikkelbroeck et al. [34].

androgen secretion by increasing the glucocorticoid dose can restore ovulation in CAH patients, in both non-classical [25] as well as classical patients [10, 31]. In some patients adequate suppression of androgen levels was not sufficient to correct menstrual abnormalities. In these patients, increased levels of progestins (progesterone and 17-hydroxyprogesterone) as a result of adrenal overproduction, interfered with normal menstrual cycling [6, 9, 32–34] (fig. 2).

The observation that hyperandrogenism in some CAH females was not suppressible by glucococorticoids led to the theory of an ovarian source of hyperandrogenism in these patients, isolated [35] or combined [36] with adrenal hyperandrogenism. The prevalence of polycystic ovaries in CAH females varies greatly [9, 36, 37]. The authors presenting the largest study of female CAH patients and their relatives concluded that the underlying lesion causing polycystic ovaries was likely to be unrelated to CAH [38, 39]. In contrast to the higher prevalence of testicular adrenal rest tumors in males, ovarian adrenal rest tumors are rare in the female CAH population [40, 41].

Besides endocrine factors, the effects of genital surgery may play a role in impaired fertility in CAH females. Reduced clitoral sensitivity or vaginal stenosis may prevent comfortable intercourse and patients own doubts about genital appearance and the function of the vagina may lead to avoidance of sexual activity [42].

Another factor may be gender atypical behavior and low maternal feelings. In some studies an increased bi/homosexual orientation is reported in CAH females [43], although in other reports this has been questioned. A review of reports on sexual orientation of women with CAH showed that the studies were heterogeneous concerning methodology and patient selection, which might explain conflicting results [44].

Fertility in Males

Reports on child rate in CAH males are rare. Jaaskeläinen et al. [45] found a child rate of 0.07 in the complete Finnish male CAH population, compared with 0.34 in age-matched Finnish males. Other authors reported parenthood only as additional information in smaller and selected patient populations, with a combined reported paternity in 22 of 103 (21%) patients studied [46–48].

The results from semen analysis are more frequently reported, but usually only in a subgroup of the study population. Taking the results of 3 larger studies together, 80 of the 100 patients agreed to provide semen for analysis. Of these 80 patients, only 19 (24%) had normal semen quality [47–49].

Causes of Subfertility in CAH Males

The most frequently reported cause of subfertility in CAH males is the presence of adrenal rest tumors in the testes [47, 48, 50]. These tumors may interfere directly (mechanically or paracrine) or indirectly (endocrine) with testicular function [51, 52]. Subfertility can also be caused by gonadotropin deficiency due to suppression of the hypothalamo-pituitary-gonadal axis by adrenal androgens (both directly and after conversion to estrogens) [53, 54].

Testicular Tumors

The reported prevalence of testicular adrenal rest tumors varies between 0 and 94% [45, 46, 48–50], strongly dependent on patient selection (prepubertal, adolescent or adult), and on the method of tumor detection (physical examination or imaging techniques) (fig. 3). Urban et al. [46] found no testicular tumors by physical examination in 30 adult patients, whereas in 3 reports using ultrasonography [45, 48, 49] testicular adrenal rest tumors were reported in 27/49 postpubertal and adult patients. Tumors have also been reported in pre-puberty [50, 55].

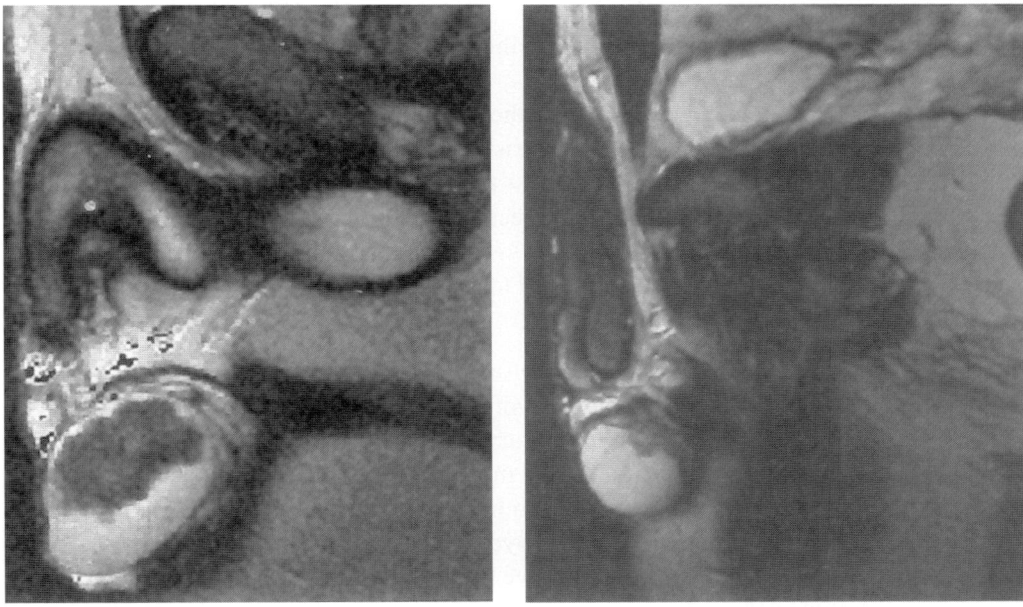

Fig. 3. Testicular adrenal rest tumors. Left: Large testicular adrenal rest tumor in a 23-year-old patient with CAH. T2-weighted MR image shows a large lobulated intratesticular mass that is hypointense compared with normal testicular parenchyma. Right: Small testicular adrenal rest tumor in an 18-year-old patient with CAH. T2-weighted MR image shows three small intratesticular masses that are hypointense compared with normal testicular parenchyma. According to Stikkelbroeck et al. [65].

Histologically, the testicular tumors in CAH patients resemble Leydig cell tumors, and differentiation can be difficult [56]. Some differences exist, however: testicular tumors associated with CAH are bilateral in 83% of the cases, Leydig cell tumors are bilateral in only 3% of cases. Malignant degeneration has not been reported in testicular tumors associated with CAH, but it occurs in 10% of Leydig cell tumors in adults. In addition, the tumors are located in the mediastinum testis, and often decrease in size when ACTH levels are suppressed by increasing the glucocorticoid dose [28, 52, 57–60].

Based on their steroid-producing properties and on the histopathology, these testicular tumors are considered to consist of ectopic adrenal tissue, which responds with hyperplasia on ACTH stimulation. Therefore the testicular tumors in CAH males are often called 'adrenal rest tumors'.

Physical examination reveals only a small proportion of all testicular tumors in CAH, depending on their size. For more accurate detection of these tumors, imaging techniques such as ultrasound or MR are required. Ultrasonography is considered the method of first choice to screen for testicular adrenal rest tumors [61].

Intensifying glucocorticoid therapy is the preferred treatment for testicular tumors in CAH [60, 62]. By increasing the glucocorticoid dose, ACTH secretion is suppressed and the adrenal rest tissue is no longer stimulated. The need for tumor shrinkage and the side effects of increasing glucocorticoid therapy must be carefully balanced, especially in asymptomatic cases [62, 63]. Increasing the glucocorticoid dose can also lead to improvement in semen quality.

Secondary Hypogonadotropism

In male patients with 21-hydroxylase deficiency adrenal androgens may suppress the hypothalamo-pituitary-gonadal axis both directly and after conversion to estrogens, and thereby may lead to hypogonadotropic hypogonadism and azoospermia [29, 48, 54]. So hypogonadotropic hypogonadism may occur in males with undiagnosed 21-hydroxylase deficiency or as a result of poor adrenal control. Some reports have shown that hypogonadism may be reversible after intensifying glucocorticoid therapy [28, 57, 59].

Prevention of Subfertility in CAH

Although fertility in CAH, both in men and women, gets only medical attention at an adult age, a more preventive strategy could be preferred.

Prevention of testicular adrenal rest tumors, the main cause of male subfertility, should already start in childhood years, since the current theories suggest that prolonged undertreatment is an important cause of tumor development. Thus, optimal hormonal control is important to prevent male infertility.

Second, early detection of tumors is important to adjust glucocorticoid therapy. It is suggested to perform routine scrotal ultrasound certainly starting from puberty onwards [64].

In females menstrual irregularities, amenorrhea and anovulation due to overproduction of adrenal androgens and progestins can already be present from early pubertal years on, and the paediatric endocrinologist should be aware of it and aim at a therapeutic regimen not only intended to momentaneous control, but also to prevent future dysregulation of fertility.

So, although fertility in CAH seems mainly an adult item, it already has to be a point of concern in childhood years. This means that childhood and adult goals of treatment in CAH cannot simply be separated but that a continuum of care must be organised for these patients. Adult treatment goals must already be implemented in childhood years with the goal of achieving fertility in later life.

References

1 White PC, Speiser PW: Congenital adrenal hyperplasia due to 21-hydroxylase deficiency. Endocr Rev 2000;21:245–291.
2 Tanner JM, Whitehouse R: Longitudinal standards for height, weight-height, height velocity and stages of puberty. Arch Dis Childh 1976;51:170–179.
3 Balsamo A, Cicognani A, Baldazzi L, Barbaro M, Baronio F, Gennari M, Bal M, Cassio A, Kontaxaki K, Cacciari E: CYP21 genotype, adult height, and prepubertal development in 55 patients treated for 21-hydroxylase deficiency. J Clin Endocrinol Metab 2003;88:5680–5688.
4 Van der Kamp HJ, Otten BJ, Buitenweg N, Muinck Keizer–Schrama de SMPF, Oostdijk W, Jansen M, Delemarre-de Waal HA, Vulsma T, Wit JM: Longitudinal analysis of growth and puberty in 21-hydroxylase deficiency patients in the Netherlands during the last 2 decades. Arch Dis Childh 2002;146:246–249.
5 Muirhead S, Sellers EAC, Guyda H: Indicators of adult height outcome in classical 21-hydroxylase deficiency congenital adrenal hyperplasia. J Pediatr 2002;141:247–252.
6 Helleday J, Siwers B, Ritzen EM, et al: Subnormal androgen and elevated progesterone levels in women treated for congenital virilizing 21-hydroxylase deficiency. J Clin Endocrinol Metab 1993;76:933–936.
7 Kuhnle U, Bullinger M, Schwarz HP: The quality of life in adult female patients with congenital adrenal hyperplasia: A comprehensive study of the impact of genital malformations and chronic disease on female patients life. Eur J Pediatr 1995;154:708–716.
8 Premawardhana LD, Hughes IA, Read GF, et al: Longer term outcome in females with congenital adrenal hyperplasia (CAH): The Cardiff experience. Clin Endocrinol Oxf 1997;46:327–332.
9 Holmes-Walker DJ, Conway GS, Honour JW, et al: Menstrual disturbance and hypersecretion of progesterone in women with congenital adrenal hyperplasia due to 21-hydroxylase deficiency. Clin Endocrinol (Oxf) 1995;43:291–296.
10 Hughes IA, Read GF: Menarche and subsequent ovarian function in girls with congenital adrenal hyperplasia. Horm Res 1982;16:100–106.
11 Yu AC, Grant DB: Adult height in women with early-treated congenital adrenal hyperplasia (21-hydroxylase type): Relation to body mass index in earlier childhood. Acta Paediatr 1995;84: 899–903.
12 Hagenfeldt K, Ritzen EM, Ringertz H, et al: Bone mass and body composition of adult women with congenital virilizing 21-hydroxylase deficiency after glucocorticoid treatment since infancy. Eur J Endocrinol 2000;143:667–671.
13 Hargitai G, Sólyom J, Battelino T, Lebl J, Pribilincová Z, Hauspie R, Kovács J, Waldhauser F, Frisch H, the MEWPE-CAH Study Group: Growth patterns and final height in congenital adrenal hyperplasia due to classical 21-hydroxylase deficiency. Horm Res 2001;55:161–171.
14 Eugster EA, DiMeglio L, Wright JC, Freidemberg GR, Sesbadri R, Pescovitz OH: Height outcome in congenital adrenal hyperplasia caused by 21-hydroxylase deficiency: A meta-analysis. J Pediatr 2001;138:26–32.
15 Jaaskelainen J, Voutilainen R: Growth of patients with 21-hydroxylase deficiency: An analysis of the factors influencing adult height. Pediatr Res 1997;41:30–33.
16 Brook CG, Zachmann M, Prader A, Murset G: Experience with long-term therapy in congenital adrenal hyperplasia. J Pediatr 1974;85:12–19.
17 Stikkelbroeck MML, Van 't Hof-Grootenboer, BAE, Hermus ARMM, Otten BJ, Van 't Hof MA: Growth inhibition by glucocorticoid treatment in salt wasting 21-hydroxylase deficiency in early infancy and in puberty. J Clin Endocrinol Metab 2003;88:3525–3530.
18 Pesccovitz OH, Comite F, Cassorla F, Dwyer AJ, Poth MA, Sperling MA, Hench K, McNemar A, Skerda M, Loriaux DL: True precocious puberty complicating congenital adrenal hyperplasia:

Treatment with a luteinizing hormone-releasing hormone analog. J Clin Endocrinol Metab 1984;58:857–861.
19 Soliman AT, AlLamki M, AlSalmi I, Asfour M: Congenital adrenal hyperplasia complicated by central precocious puberty: Linear growth during infancy and treatment with gonadotropin-releasing hormone analog. Metabolism 1997;46:513–517.
20 Quintos JBQ, Vogiatzi MG, Harbison MD, New MI: Growth hormone therapy alone or in combination with gonadotropin-releasing hormone analog therapy to improve the height deficit in children with congenital adrenal hyperplasia. J Clin Endocrinol Metab 2001;86:1511–1517.
21 Mulaikal RM, Migeon CJ, Rock JA: Fertility rates in female patients with congenital adrenal hyperplasia due to 21-hydroxylase deficiency. N Engl J Med 1987;316:178–182.
22 Federman DD: Psychosexual adjustment in congenital adrenal hyperplasia. N Engl J Med 1987;316:209–211.
23 Jaaskelainen J, Hippelainen M, Kiekara O, et al: Child rate, pregnancy outcome and ovarian function in females with classical 21-hydroxylase deficiency. Acta Obstet Gynecol Scand 2000;79:687–692.
24 Krone N, Wachter I, Stefanidou M, et al: Mothers with congenital adrenal hyperplasia and their children: Outcome of pregnancy, birth and childhood. Clin Endocrinol (Oxf) 2001;55:523–529.
25 Feldman S, Billaud L, Thalabard JC, et al: Fertility in women with late-onset adrenal hyperplasia due to 21-hydroxylase deficiency. J Clin Endocrinol Metab 1992;74:635–639.
26 Birnbaum MD, Rose LI: Late onset adrenocortical hydroxylase deficiencies associated with menstrual dysfunction. Obstet Gynecol 1984;63:445–451.
27 Augarten A, Weissenberg R, Pariente C, et al: Reversible male infertility in late onset congenital adrenal hyperplasia. J Endocrinol Invest 1991;14:237–240.
28 Wischusen J, Baker HW, Hudson B: Reversible male infertility due to congenital adrenal hyperplasia. Clin Endocrinol (Oxf) 1981;14:571–577.
29 Bonaccorsi AC, Adler I, Figueiredo JG: Male infertility due to congenital adrenal hyperplasia: Testicular biopsy findings, hormonal evaluation, and therapeutic results in three patients. Fertil Steril 1987;47:664–670.
30 Cabrera MS, Vogiatzi MG, New MI: Long term outcome in adult males with classic congenital adrenal hyperplasia. J Clin Endocrinol Metab 2001;86:3070–3078.
31 Richards GE, Grumbach MM, Kaplan SL, et al: The effect of long acting glucocorticoids on menstrual abnormalities in patients with virilizing congenital adrenal hyperplasia. J Clin Endocrinol Metab 1978;47:1208–1215.
32 Rosenfield RL, Bickel S, Razdan AK: Amenorrhea related to progestin excess in congenital adrenal hyperplasia. Obstet Gynecol 1980;56:208–215.
33 Riad-Fahmy D, Read GF, Walker RF, et al: Steroids in saliva for assessing endocrine function. Endocr Rev 1982;3:367–395.
34 Stikkelbroeck MML, Sweep CGJ, Braat DDM, Hermus ARMM, Otten BJ: Menstrual cycles, ovulation and adrenal suppression, monitored by saliva sampling in female patients with 21-hydroxylase deficiency. Fertil Steril 2003;80:1030–1036.
35 Barnes RB, Rosenfield RL, Ehrmann DA, et al: Ovarian hyperandrogynism as a result of congenital adrenal virilizing disorders: Evidence for perinatal masculinization of neuroendocrine function in women. J Clin Endocrinol Metab 1994;79:1328–1333.
36 Ghizzoni L, Virdis R, Vottero A, et al: Pituitary-ovarian responses to leuprolide acetate testing in patients with congenital adrenal hyperplasia due to 21-hydroxylase deficiency. J Clin Endocrinol Metab 1996;81:601–606.
37 Levin JH, Carmina E, Lobo RA: Is the inappropriate gonadotropin secretion of patients with polycystic ovary syndrome similar to that of patients with adult-onset congenital adrenal hyperplasia? Fertil Steril 1991;56:635–640.
38 Hague WM, Adams J, Rodda C, et al: The prevalence of polycystic ovaries in patients with congenital adrenal hyperplasia and their close relatives. Clin Endocrinol (Oxf) 1990;33:501–510.
39 Hague WM, Adams J, Algar V, et al: HLA associations in patients with polycystic ovaries and in patients with congenital adrenal hyperplasia caused by 21-hydroxylase deficiency. Clin Endocrinol (Oxf) 1990;32:407–415.
40 Russo G, Paesano P, Taccagni G, et al: Ovarian adrenal-like tissue in congenital adrenal hyperplasia. N Engl J Med 1998;339:853–854.

41 Al Ahmadie HA, Stanek J, Liu J, et al: Ovarian 'tumor' of the adrenogenital syndrome: The first reported case. Am J Surg Pathol 2001;25:1443–1450.
42 Krege S, Walz KH, Hauffa BP, et al: Long-term follow-up of female patients with congenital adrenal hyperplasia from 21-hydroxylase deficiency, with special emphasis on the results of vaginoplasty. BJU Int 2000;86:253–258.
43 Meyer-Bahlburg HFL: Gender and sexuality in classic congenital adrenal hyperplasia. Endocrinol Metab Clin N Am 2001;30:155–171,VIII.
44 Zucker KJ, Bradley SJ, Oliver G, et al: Psychosexual development of women with congenital adrenal hyperplasia. Horm Behav 1996;30:300–318.
45 Jaaskelainen J, Kiekara O, Hippelainen M, Voutilainen R: Pituitary gonadal axis and child rate in males with classical 21-hydroxylase deficiency. J Endocrinol Invest 2000;23:23–27.
46 Urban MD, Lee PA, Migeon CJ: Adult height and fertility in men with congenital virilizing adrenal hyperplasia. N Engl J Med 1978;299:1392–1396.
47 Wuesthof AR, Willig RP, Schulze W, Hoepffner W, Knorr D, Schwarz HP: Spermatogenesis is impaired in men with congenital adrenal hyperplasia. Horm Res 1998;50:104–104.
48 Cabrera MS, Vogiatzi MG, New MI: Long term outcome in adult males with classic congenital adrenal hyperplasia. J Clin Endocrinol Metab 2001;86:3070–3078.
49 Stikkelbroeck NMML, Otten BJ, Pasic A, Jager GJ, Sweep CGJ, Noordam K, Hermus ARMM: High prevalence of testicular adrenal rest tumors, impaired spermatogenesis, and Leydig cell failure in adolescent and adult males with congenital adrenal hyperplasia. J Clin Endocrinol Metab 2001;86:5721–5728.
50 Avila NA, Premkumar A, Shawker TH, Jones JV, Laue L, Cutler GB: Testicular adrenal rest tissue in congenital adrenal hyperplasia: Findings at gray-scale and color Doppler US. Radiology 1996;198:99–104.
51 Cutfield RG, Bateman JM, Odell WD: Infertility caused by bilateral testicular masses secondary to congenital adrenal hyperplasia (21-hydroxylase deficiency). Fertil Steril 1983;40:809–814.
52 Cunnah D, Perry L, Dacie JA, Grant DB, Lowe DG, Savage MO, Besser GM: Bilateral testicular tumours in congenital adrenal hyperplasia: A continuing diagnostic and therapeutic dilemma. Clin Endocrinol (Oxf) 1989;30:141–147.
53 Bonaccorsi AC, Adler I, Figueiredo JG: Male infertility due to congenital adrenal hyperplasia: Testicular biopsy findings, hormonal evaluation, and therapeutic results in three patients. Fertil Steril 1987;47:664–670.
54 Moore GW, Lacroix A, Rabin D, McKenna TJ: Gonadal dysfunction in adult men with congenital adrenal hyperplasia. Acta Endocrinol (Copenh) 1980;95:185–193.
55 Shanklin DR, Richardson AP Jr, Rothstein G: Testicular hilar nodules in adrenogenital syndrome. Am J Dis Child 1963;106:243–250.
56 Rich MA, Keating MA: Leydig cell tumors and tumors associated with congenital adrenal hyperplasia. Urol Clin N Am 2000;27:519–528,X.
57 Kim I, Young RH, Scully RE: Leydig cell tumors of the testis. A clinicopathological analysis of 40 cases and review of the literature. Am J Surg Pathol 1985;9:177–192.
58 Knudsen JL, Savage A, Mobb GE: The testicular 'tumour' of adrenogenital syndrome–a persistent diagnostic pitfall. Histopathology 1991;19:468–470.
59 Augarten A, Weissenberg R, Pariente C, Sack J: Reversible male infertility in late onset congenital adrenal hyperplasia. J Endocrinol Invest 1991;14:237–240.
60 Rutgers JL, Young RH, Scully RE: The testicular tumor of the adrenogenital syndrome: A report of six cases and review of the literature on testicular masses in patients with adrenocortical disorders. Am J Surg Pathol 1988;12:503–513.
61 Avila NA, Premkumar A, Merke DP: Testicular adrenal rest tissue in congenital adrenal hyperplasia: Comparison of MR imaging and sonographic findings. Am J Roentgenol 1999;172:1003–1006.
62 Walker BR, Skoog SJ, Winslow BH, Canning DA, Tank ES: Testis sparing surgery for steroid unresponsive testicular tumors of the adrenogenital syndrome. J Urol 1997;157:1460–1463.
63 Stikkelbroeck MML, Hermus ARMM, Suliman HM, Jager JG, Otten BJ: Asymptomatic testicular adrenal rest tumours in adolescent and adult males with congenital adrenal hyperplasia: Basal and follow-up investigation after 2.6 years. J Pediatr Endocrinol Metab 2004;17:645–653.

64 Hughes I: Asymptomatic testicular adrenal rest tumours. J Pediatr Endocrinol Metab 2004;17: 589–590.
65 Stikkelbroeck MML, Suliman HM, Otten BJ, Hermus ARMM, Blickman JG, Jager GJ: Testicular adrenal rest tumours in postpubertal males with congenital adrenal hyperplasia: Sonographic and MR features. Eur Radiol 2003;13:1597–1603.

Dr. Barto J. Otten
Department of Pediatric Endocrinology, University Hospital St. Radboud
Postbus 9101, NL-6500 HB Nijmegen (The Netherlands)
Tel. +31 24 361 44 29, Fax +31 24 361 91 23, E-Mail b.otten@cukz.umcn.nl

Delemarre-van de Waal HA (ed): Abnormalities in Puberty. Scientific and Clinical Advances.
Endocr Dev. Basel, Karger, 2005, vol 8, pp 67–80

Molecular Genetics of Isolated Hypogonadotropic Hypogonadism and Kallmann Syndrome

Beate Karges[a], *Nicolas de Roux*[b]

[a] University Children's Hospital, University of Ulm, Ulm, Germany;
[b] INSERM U584, Hormone Targets, Medical Faculty Necker-Enfants Malades, and University Paris XI, Paris, France

Abstract

Isolated hypogonadotropic hypogonadism (IHH) is characterized by complete or partial failure of pubertal development due to impaired secretion of luteinizing hormone (LH) and follicle-stimulating hormone (FSH). In the molecular pathogenesis of IHH, the gonadotropin-releasing hormone receptor (GnRH-R) and associated proteins have evolved as a central element. GnRH-R germline mutations were among the first genetic alterations identified in patients with IHH. These mutations are associated with impaired GnRH binding, ligand-induced signal transduction, or both, leading to various degrees of LH and FSH deficiency. As GnRH-R mutations explain several but not all cases of IHH, the search for new candidate genes continued in informative families. In 2003, mutations of the KiSS-1-derived peptide receptor GPR54 were identified in patients with IHH, opening a new pathway in the physiologic regulation of puberty and reproduction. GPR54 is putatively involved in the control of GnRH secretion. IHH associated with impaired olfactory function (Kallmann syndrome) may be caused by mutations of the X-chromosomal KAL1 (encoding anosmin) or the fibroblast growth factor receptor 1 genes (FGFR1), both leading to agenesis of olfactory and GnRH-secreting neurons. In addition to their clinical and diagnostic value, the identification of genetic and functional alterations in IHH helps to unravel the complex regulation of the gonadotropic axis.

Hypothalamic gonadotropin-releasing hormone (GnRH) plays a key role in induction of gonadotropin secretion from the anterior pituitary. A disturbed GnRH function may result from a lack of neuronal migration, defective synthesis and secretion of GnRH or inactivating mutations of the GnRH receptor

(GnRH-R). In recent years the identification of disease-associated gene mutations in affected patients, and the subsequent characterization of altered gene function provided new insights in the regulation of puberty and reproduction [1–4].

Among monogenetic disorders of delayed puberty and human reproductive disease [5–8] we will here focus on recent advances in GnRH release and action causing idiopathic isolated hypogonadotropic hypogonadism (IHH) and Kallmann syndrome. The novel identification of inactivating mutations in the fibroblast growth factor receptor 1 (FGFR1/ KAL2) gene [9, 10] leading to GnRH deficiency added new information on the regulation of olfactory and GnRH neuron migration. Comprehensive studies of GnRH resistance due to inactivation of the GnRH-R function could explain the phenotypic variation in several clinical cases of IHH [3]. However, GnRH-R variants does not explain all cases of IHH and very recently, inactivating mutations in the G protein-coupled receptor 54 (GPR 54) were found in affected individuals [4, 11], delineating new mechanisms in the pathogenesis of hypogonadotropic hypogonadism.

G Protein-Coupled Receptors in IHH

The receptors for GnRH-R, gonadotropins (luteinizing hormone (LH) and follicle-stimulating hormone (FSH)) and the GPR54 belong to the family of G protein-coupled receptors (GPCRs), a universal receptor system with sequence homology to the light receptor rhodopsin [12]. More than 1,000 different GPCRs serve as receptors for a large number of various ligands involved in intercellular communication, thus explaining their high conservation during evolution in most species [13].

Type A GPCRs are characterized by several common features, including seven transmembrane spanning domains, connected by three alternating intracellular and extracellular loops (fig. 1) [14]. Several amino acid residues are highly conserved within these receptors, suggesting that these positions are critical for receptor function [12]. Specific peptidic ligand binding takes place at the N-terminal extracellular domain or extracellular loops leading to sequential conformational changes that transduce the receptor to its active state. The initiation of intracellular signalling cascades is mediated by the activation of membrane-bound G-protein, leading to specific gene expression and cell functions, e.g. gonadotropin hormone synthesis and secretion in anterior pituitary cells.

Several disease causing mutations that affect the gonadotropic axis have been identified in GPCRs and their ligands [3–6, 11]. The functional consequences of disease-associated GPCR structure can be successfully studied in

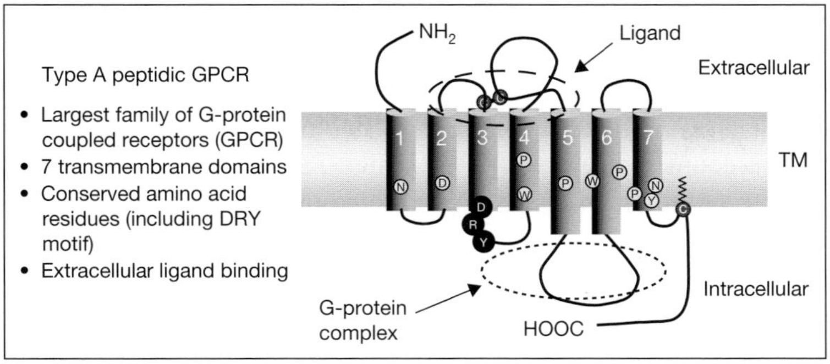

Fig. 1. G protein-coupled receptors (GPCR), type A: a common target of disease-associated mutations in hypogonadotropic hypogonadism. In the GnRH-receptor, the DRY motif is replaced by DRS (Asp-Arg-Ser).

silico by molecular modelling, a strategy based on the crystallography co-ordinates of rhodopsin, a prototypic type A GPCR [2].

GnRH and GnRH-R Structure

GnRH (synonym: luteinizing hormone-releasing hormone, LHRH) is synthesized by hypothalamic neurons and secreted in a pulsatile fashion into the pituitary portal circulation [15]. Binding of GnRH to high-affinity receptors in cell membranes of gonadotropes in the anterior pituitary induces synthesis and release of LH and FSH. Pathogenic mechanisms causing isolated hypogonadotropic hypogonadism may affect synthesis or secretion of hypothalamic GnRH and function of the GnRH receptor. As a consequence, in the GnRH-R system both ligand and receptor have been analyzed as candidate genes in the context of isolated hypogonadotropic hypogonadism.

After identification of the hypogonadal mouse (*hpg* mouse) carrying a GnRH gene deletion [16], the GnRH gene was considered a promising candidate for mutational analysis in patients with idiopathic hypogonadotropic hypogonadism (IHH). In affected individuals, deficient hypothalamic GnRH or impaired GnRH action was postulated because exogenous GnRH was able to stimulate gonadotropin secretion [17]. The human GnRH gene, located on 8p21–p11.2, comprises 3 exons, encoding a protein of 92 amino acids [18]. The decapetide GnRH is preceded by a signal peptide of 23 amino acids and cleaved from its precursor protein. However, no mutations of the human GnRH gene have been identified so far in patients with IHH (OMIM 152760) [19–21].

The receptor for GnRH (GnRH-R) was initially not considered as the candidate gene for patients with idiopathic hypogonadotropic hypogonadism (IHH), as exogenous GnRH administration could induce release of gonadotropins LH and FSH. The evidence of partial loss-of-function mutations in other G protein-coupled receptors (GPCRs) like TSH-R [22, 23] and LH-R [24, 25] associated with human diseases finally led to the discovery of inactivating GnRH-R mutations causing IHH in patients with a normal response to exogenous GnRH [1]. The human GnRH-R gene is localized on chromosome 4q21.2, comprises 3 exons, encoding a protein of 328 amino acids [26]. The GnRH-R has several unique features compared to other type A GPCRs, including the lack of an intracellular C-terminal domain [27] and replacement of the conserved DRY motif in transmembrane domain 3 by DRS (Asp-Arg-Ser). Activation of the GnRH-R by ligand binding results in intracellular activation of phospholipase C and mitogen-activated protein kinase (MAPK) cascades and regulates gonadotropin transcription and secretion [28, 29].

GnRH-R Gene Structure and Function in IHH

Inactivating germline mutations of the GnRH-R were identified in several patients with hypogonadotropic hypogonadism (OMIM 138850), equally affecting male and female individuals [1, 2, 30–40]. In familial cases of normosmic IHH whose pedigrees suggested autosomal-recessive transmission, in 40% of patients a mutated GnRH-R was found, while only 12% of sporadic cases of IHH were associated with GnRH-R variants [36]. These GnRH-R mutations are predominantly missense mutations and only two nonsense mutations and one intron mutation were described [3]. Until now, 18 different human substitutions of the GnRH-R gene were reported. The GnRH-R mutations are distributed widely throughout the protein (fig. 2) but two 'hot spots', the Q106R and R262Q substitutions are frequently found in affected individuals. Patients with IHH due to GnRH-R mutations are either homozygous for an inactivating substitution or compound heterozygous for two different mutations.

In vitro studies of natural GnRH-R substitutions revealed GnRH-R inactivation by reduced or absent ligand binding and signal transduction for all GnRH-R mutations identified so far [3, 39, 40]. The molecular mechanism for loss of receptor function may result from disturbed intracellular processing [37, 41–45] and the GnRH-R mutant may even exhibit a dominant negative effect with retention of the wild-type GnRH-R in the endoplasmatic reticulum in vitro [45]. However, heterozygous individuals carrying a dominant negative GnRH-R mutant do not present any specific phenotype. The loss of GnRH-R function may also result from specific inactivation in receptors normally

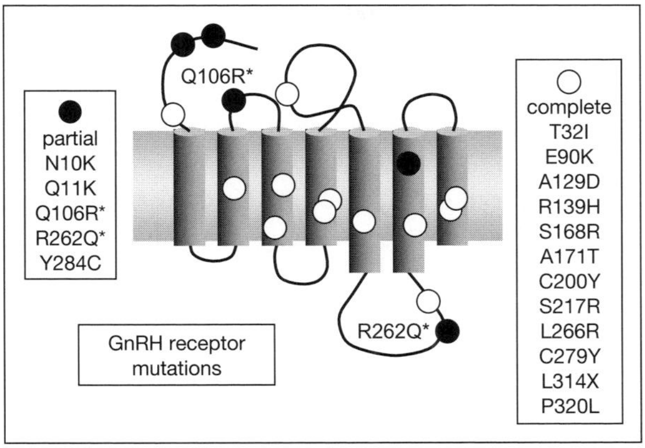

Fig. 2. Mutations of the GnRH-receptor (GnRH-R) as a cause of hypogonadotropic hypogonadism. Mutations associated with complete (open symbols) or partial (black symbols) loss of GnRH-R function. *Most frequently identified GnRH-R mutations.

expressed at the cell surface [2, 32]. For example, the introduction of an additional hydrogen bond in the GnRH-R variant A171T has been shown to stabilize the GnRH-R in an inactive conformation, thus preventing receptor activation by the natural ligand [2].

Correlation of GnRH-R Genotype and Phenotype

In vivo and in vitro studies of GnRH-R substitutions distinguish between complete or partial loss of receptor function [3]. The combination of GnRH-R substitutions on both alleles determine the clinical phenotype in affected patients. Clinical severity of GnRH-R inactivation may thus be correlated to the GnRH-R genotype. While patients homozygous for a partially inactivating GnRH-R mutation present with partial hypogonadism [46, 47] like fertile eunuch syndrome, patients with complete inactivating GnRH-R variants on both alleles present with severe hypogonadism [32, 35, 36, 38, 48, 49]. GnRH administration in the context of GnRH testing may overcome partially inactive GnRH receptors and result in normal response to GnRH with increase of gonadotropins. Comparison of compound heterozygous with homozygous patients suggests that the phenotype is mainly determined by the GnRH-R variant with the less severe loss of function.

Identification of GnRH-R mutations may further guide fertility treatment in affected patients as they are mostly resistant to pulsatile GnRH treatment.

While repeated exposure to high doses of pulsatile GnRH may result in some response inducing ovulation in patients with partially inactivating GnRH-R variants [46, 50], individuals with complete inactivating GnRH-R mutations do not respond to GnRH treatment [32, 51] but to therapeutic administration of gonadotropins.

Comparison between patients carrying the same GnRH-R variant revealed inter-individual phenotypic variation even within the same family [31, 33, 52]. These phenotypic differences in patients with identical GnRH-R mutations are probably modified by other genes involved in gonadotrope function.

The KISS-1-Derived Peptide Receptor GPR54

The genetic heterogeneity in IHH suggested involvement of so far undiscovered proteins in the regulation of gonadotropic function [4, 15, 21, 53]. Linkage analysis in informative families with recessive normosmic IHH confirmed the presence of further genes encoding proteins playing a major role in the gonadotropic axis and therefore pathogenesis of IHH [4, 54].

By homozygosity whole genome mapping [55] in a consanguineous family with IHH, a new locus within the short arm of chromosome 19 (19p) was identified [4, 54]. Several genes localized within this region are putatively involved in onset of puberty and were thus considered potential candidate [56, 57]. Finally, inactivating mutations of GPR54 were identified in affected patients [4, 11]. The gene of the G protein-coupled receptor GPR54 is located on chromosome 19p13.3, comprises 5 exons, encoding a protein of 398 amino acids [58]. The GPR54 receptor has typical features of type A GPCRs (fig. 3) and is expressed in human brain (hypothalamus), pituitary gland and placenta [59, 60].

The phenotype observed in GPR54$^{-/-}$ mouse is characterized by hypogonadism in male and female mice with low plasma levels for LH and FSH [11]. GnRH administration led to an increase in LH and FSH plasma levels suggesting persistent expression of the GnRH-R in membranes of gonadotrope cells of GPR54$^{-/-}$ mice. The observation that hypothalamic concentration of GnRH in GPR54$^{-/-}$ mice was not different from wild-type mice is in favor with a role of GPR54 function for modulation of GnRH secretion. The natural ligand of the GPR54 is the KISS-1-derived peptide. Intracerebral and peripheral injection of kisspeptins led to a significant increase of LH and FSH in mouse and rat [61–63] confirming that the KISS-1-peptide GPR54 signalling regulates hypothalamic secretion of GnRH.

KISS-1-derived peptide, the ligand of GPR54, was initially identified as a human metastasis suppressor gene in melanomas and breast carcinomas [64].

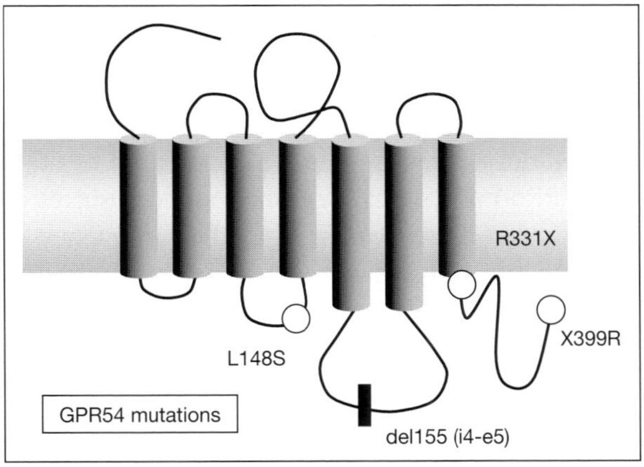

Fig. 3. Inactivating mutations of the GPR54 identified in patients with isolated hypogonadotropic hypogonadism.

The KISS-1 gene is located on 1q32–q41 and comprises 3 exons encoding a protein of 145 amino acids. Recently [65] it was demonstrated that a KISS-1-derived protein of 54 amino acids isolated from human placenta is the endogenous ligand of the orphan GPR54. This truncated form of KISS-1 was named metastin. The role of the 54 amino acid peptide for regulation of puberty was opened with the discovery of inactivating mutations in its receptor GPR54 in patients with hypogonadotropic hypogonadism [4, 11, 57]. The KISS-1 gene and their encoded proteins are now promising candidates to be investigated in the context of pubertal development and reproduction.

GPR54 Mutations in IHH

So far four different natural occurring human mutations were described in patients with IHH and recessive inheritance equally affecting male and female patients (fig. 3, OMIM 604161). These mutations were homozygous deletion, missense and nonsense mutations [4, 11] of the GPR54 gene. Inactivation of the GPR54 gene as a cause of human hypogonadotropic hypogonadism was confirmed by functional studies in vitro and in a GPR54-deficient mouse model [11, 66].

The clinical phenotype in patients with inactivating substitutions of the GPR54 include hypogonadism with small testes (1–4 ml), sparse pubic hair and a penis length of 7 cm in affected males [4, 21]. In a female patient partial hypogonadism with spontaneous breast development and a single uterine bleeding was reported. All patients had retarded bone age and normal sense of smell. Hormonal measurements revealed low plasma testosterone or estradiol levels, respectively, with low plasma levels of gonadotropins but blunted response to exogenous GnRH [4, 11, 21]. In one patient, low-amplitude pulses of LH were measured with a leftward-shifted dose-response curve as compared to other patients with IHH but without GPR54 mutation, suggesting reduced secretion of GnRH and high sensitivity to exogenous GnRH [11]. The frequency of GPR54 mutations among patients with IHH is low, being approximately 1–2% in total cases of IHH [4, 11, 57]. Therefore, further and so far undiscovered mechanisms in the pathogenesis of IHH have to be identified.

Kallmann Syndrome

The genetic nature of hypogonadism associated with the inability to smell (anosmia) was postulated by Kallmann et al. [67] in 1944 and described as 'olfactogenital dysplasia' by de Morsier [68] in 1954. Kallmann syndrome results from a defect in migration of olfactory nerves and GnRH neurons [69]. Affected individuals typically present with congenital isolated gonadotropin deficiency and anosmia or hyposmia. Although this disease is genetically heterogeneous with reports indicating autosomal-dominant, recessive and X-linked transmission, only the latter was understood at the molecular level after identification of mutations in the KAL1 gene [10, 70–74]. The KAL1 gene is localized at Xp22.3, comprises 14 exons encoding the glycoprotein anosmin1 of 680 amino acids. Anosmin plays a key role in migration of GnRH neurons and olfactory nerves to the hypothalamus [75, 76]. Several types of KAL1 gene abnormalities were identified in patients with Kallmann syndrome (OMIM 308700). They include missense and nonsense mutations, splice site mutations, intragenic deletions and chromosomal deletions involving the entire KAL1 gene [10, 74, 77]. The phenotype in males with KAL1 mutations consists of delayed puberty and hypogonadotropic hypogonadism and variable degree of anosmia/hyposmia and may also include mirror movements and unilateral renal agenesis with clinical heterogeneity in siblings [73]. Female carriers in families with KAL1 mutations have no specific phenotype [78]. While KAL1 mutations were found in only 14% of familial X-linked and 11% of males with sporadic Kallmann syndrome, the majority of familial cases of Kallmann syndrome are caused by defects in autosomal genes [78, 79].

In 2003, Dode et al. [9] studied two sporadic cases with different contiguous gene syndromes both including Kallmann syndrome. A new candidate region within the short arm of chromosome 8 was defined for autosomal

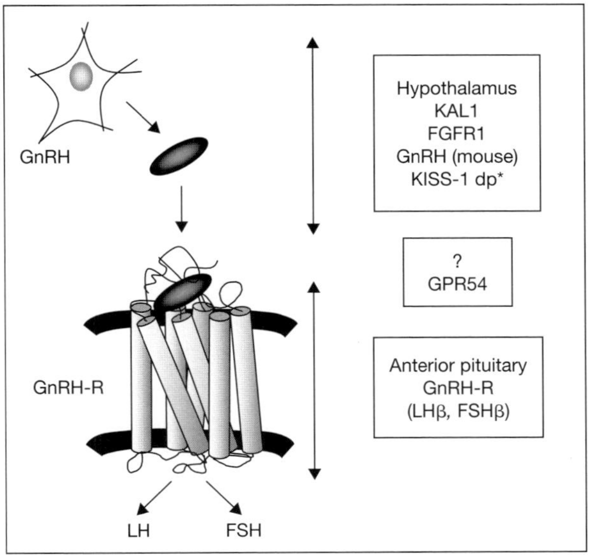

Fig. 4. Synopsis: Genetic causes of isolated hypogonadotropic hypogonadism. *Denotes KISS-1 derived peptide (dp), which acts either at the hypothalamic or the pituitary level.

Kallmann syndrome. The FGF receptor 1 gene localized within the candidate region was considered as candidate gene because FGF receptors are involved in olfactory bulb development [80, 81]. The FGFR1 gene is localized at 8p11.2–12 and comprises 18 exons coding for a protein of 822 amino acids. Several heterozygous nonsense and missense mutations and small deletions of FGFR1 (also called KAL2) were identified in familial and sporadic cases of Kallmann syndrome [9, 10]. As several mutations concern residues involved in receptor folding and signal transduction it is concluded that the inactivation of the FGF receptor 1 causes Kallmann syndrome (OMIM 136350, 147950). The frequency of FGFR1 mutations in Kallmann syndrome is approximately 10% [9, 10]. Affected individuals present with anosmia, delayed puberty, variable reproductive phenotype and may include dental agenesis and cleft palate. A high variability of phenotypic expression was observed in familial cases. It is suggested that the KAL1 gene product anosmin1 is involved in regulation of FGF function. While mutations in the KAL1 and FGFR1 genes could delineate the disease causing mechanisms in several patients with Kallmann syndrome, the genetic source of this disease remains to be determined in cases with recessive forms of Kallmann syndrome (KAL3, OMIM 244200) and in affected individuals without mutations in the KAL1 or FGFR1/KAL2 genes.

Conclusion

The recognition of inactivating germline mutations in patients with isolated hypogonadotropic hypogonadism provided substantial progress in understanding the molecular pathogenesis of abnormal GnRH function (fig. 4). GnRH deficiency due to aberrant migration of GnRH and olfactory neurons is caused by inactivation of anosmin or the fibroblast growth factor receptor 1. Hypothalamic secretion of GnRH is putatively regulated by the KiSS-1-derived peptide receptor GPR54. Action of GnRH is transmitted through the GnRH-R in which amino acid substitutions result in GnRH resistance due to impaired hormone-receptor interaction. The identification of new pathways in GnRH synthesis, secretion and action added new information on the regulation of pubertal development and reproduction in humans and offer novel targets for therapeutic approaches in patients with hypogonadotropic hypogonadism.

Acknowledgement

Supported by a Clinical Fellowship Award of the Deutsche Gesellschaft für Endokrinologie APE (to B. K.).

References

1 de-Roux N, Young J, Misrahi M, Genet R, Chanson P, Schaison G, Milgrom E: A family with hypogonadotropic hypogonadism and mutations in the gonadotropin-releasing hormone receptor. N Engl J Med 1997;337:1597–1602.

2 Karges B, Karges W, Mine M, Ludwig L, Kuhne R, Milgrom E, de-Roux N: Mutation Ala(171)Thr stabilizes the gonadotropin-releasing hormone receptor in its inactive conformation, causing familial hypogonadotropic hypogonadism. J Clin Endocrinol Metab 2003;88:1873–1879.

3 Karges B, Karges W, de Roux N: Clinical and molecular genetics of the human gonadotropin releasing-hormone receptor. Hum Reprod Update 2003;9:523–530.

4 de-Roux N, Genin E, Carel JC, Matsuda F, Chaussain JL, Milgrom E: Hypogonadotropic hypogonadism due to loss of function of the KiSS1-derived peptide receptor GPR54. Proc Natl Acad Sci USA 2003;100:10972–10976.

5 Themmen APN, Huhtaniemi IT: Mutations of gonadotropins and gonadotropin receptors: Elucidating the physiology and pathophysiology of pituitary-gonadal function. Endocr Rev 2000;21:551–583.

6 de-Roux N, Milgrom E: Inherited disorders of GnRH and gonadotropin receptors. Mol Cell Endocrinol 2001;179:83–87.

7 Achermann JC, Ozisik G, Meeks JJ, Jameson JL: Genetic causes of human reproductive disease. J Clin Endocrinol Metab 2002;87:2447–2454.

8 Kalantaridou SN, Chrousos GP: Clinical review 148: Monogenic disorders of puberty. J Clin Endocrinol Metab 2002;87:2481–2494.

9 Dode C, Levilliers J, Dupont JM, et al: Loss-of-function mutations in FGFR1 cause autosomal dominant Kallmann syndrome. Nat Genet 2003;33:463–465.

10 Sato N, Katsumata N, Kagami M, et al: Clinical assessment and mutation analysis of Kallmann syndrome (KAL1) and fibroblast growth factor receptor 1 (FGFR1, or KAL2) in five families and 18 sporadic patients. J Clin Endocrinol Metab 2004;89:1079–1088.

11 Seminara SB, Messager S, Chatzidaki EE, Thresher RR, Acierno JS Jr, Shagoury JK, Bo-Abbas Y, Kuohung W, Schwinof KM, Hendrick AG, Zahn D, Dixon J, Kaiser UB, Slaugenhaupt SA, Gusella JF, O'Rahilly S, Carlton MB, Crowley WF Jr, Aparicio SA, Colledge WH: The GPR54 gene as a regulator of puberty. N Engl J Med 2003;349:1614–1627.

12 Gether U: Uncovering molecular mechanisms involved in activation of G protein-coupled receptors. Endocr Rev 2000;21:90–113.

13 Bockaert J, Pin JP: Molecular tinkering of G protein-coupled receptors: an evolutionary success. Embo J 1999;18:1723–1729.

14 Palczewski K, Kumasaka T, Hori T, Behnke CA, Motoshima H, Fox BA, Le-Trong I, Teller DC, Okada T, Stenkamp RE, Yamamoto M, Miyano M: Crystal structure of rhodopsin: A G protein-coupled receptor. Science 2000;289:739–745.

15 Seminara SB, Hayes FJ, Crowley WF: Gonadotropin-releasing hormone deficiency in the human (idiopathic hypogonadotropic hypogonadism and Kallmann's syndrome): Pathophysiological and genetic considerations. Endocr Rev 1998;19:521–539.

16 Mason AJ, Hayflick JS, Zoeller RT, Young WS 3rd, Phillips HS, Nikolics K, Seeburg PH: A deletion truncating the gonadotropin-releasing hormone gene is responsible for hypogonadism in the hpg mouse. Science 1986;234:1366–1371.

17 Waldstreicher J, Seminara SB, Jameson JL, Geyer A, Nachtigall LB, Boepple PA, Holmes LB, Crowley WF Jr: The genetic and clinical heterogeneity of gonadotropin-releasing hormone deficiency in the human. J Clin Endocrinol Metab 1996;81:4388–4395.

18 Seeburg PH, Adelman JP: Characterization of cDNA for precursor of human luteinizing hormone releasing hormone. Nature 1984;311:666–668.

19 Weiss J, Adams E, Whitcomb RW, Crowley WF Jr, Jameson JL: Normal sequence of the gonadotropin-releasing hormone gene in patients with idiopathic hypogonadotropic hypogonadism. Biol Reprod 1991;45:743–747.

20 Layman LC, Peak D, Jin M: The prevalence and potential effects of gonadotropin releasing hormone gene point mutations in idiopathic hypogonadotropic hypogonadism (abstract). Endocr Soc 1996;p3–40:855.

21 Bo-Abbas Y, Acierno JS, Shagoury JK, Crowley WF, Seminara SB: Autosomal recessive idiopathic hypogonadotropic hypogonadism: Genetic analysis excludes mutations in the gonadotropin-releasing hormone (GnRH) and GnRH receptor genes. J Clin Endocrinol Metab 2003;88:2730–2737.

22 Sunthornthepvarakui T, Gottschalk ME, Hayashi Y, Refetoff S: Brief report: Resistance to thyrotropin caused by mutations in the thyrotropin-receptor gene. N Engl J Med 1995;332:155–160.

23 de-Roux N, Misrahi M, Brauner R, Houang M, Carel JC, Granier M, Le-Bouc Y, Ghinea N, Boumedienne A, Toublanc JE, Milgrom E: Four families with loss of function mutations of the thyrotropin receptor. J Clin Endocrinol Metab 1996;81:4229–4235.

24 Latronico AC, Anasti J, Arnhold IJ, Rapaport R, Mendonca BB, Bloise W, Castro M, Tsigos C, Chrousos GP: Brief report: Testicular and ovarian resistance to luteinizing hormone caused by inactivating mutations of the luteinizing hormone-receptor gene. N Engl J Med 1996;334:507–512.

25 Laue LL, Wu SM, Kudo M, Bourdony CJ, Cutler GB Jr, Hsueh AJ, Chan WY: Compound heterozygous mutations of the luteinizing hormone receptor gene in Leydig cell hypoplasia. Mol Endocrinol 1996;10:987–997.

26 Stojilkovic SS, Reinhart J, Catt KJ: Gonadotropin-releasing hormone receptors: Structure and signal transduction pathways. Endocr Rev 1994;15:462–499.

27 Sealfon SC, Weinstein H, Millar RP: Molecular mechanisms of ligand interaction with the gonadotropin-releasing hormone receptor. Endocr Rev 1997;18:180–205.

28 Naor Z, Harris D, Shacham S: Mechanism of GnRH receptor signaling: Combinatorial cross-talk of Ca^{2+} and protein kinase C. Front Neuroendocrinol 1998;19:1–19.

29 Bedecarrats GY, Linher KD, Kaiser UB: Two common naturally occurring mutations in the human gonadotropin-releasing hormone (GnRH) receptor have differential effects on gonadotropin gene expression and on GnRH-mediated signal transduction. J Clin Endocrinol Metab 2003;88: 834–843.

30 Layman LC, Cohen DP, Jin M, Xie J, Li Z, Reindollar RH, Bolbolan S, Bick DP, Sherins RR, Duck LW, Musgrove LC, Sellers JC, Neill JD: Mutations in gonadotropin-releasing hormone receptor gene cause hypogonadotropic hypogonadism. Nat Genet 1998;18:14–15.

31 Caron P, Chauvin S, Christin-Maitre S, Bennet A, Lahlou N, Counis R, Bouchard P, Kottler ML: Resistance of hypogonadic patients with mutated GnRH receptor genes to pulsatile GnRH administration. J Clin Endocrinol Metab 1999;84:990–996.

32 Pralong FP, Gomez F, Castillo E, Cotecchia S, Abuin L, Aubert ML, Portmann L, Gaillard RC: Complete hypogonadotropic hypogonadism associated with a novel inactivating mutation of the gonadotropin-releasing hormone receptor. J Clin Endocrinol Metab 1999;84:3811–3816.

33 de-Roux N, Young J, Brailly-Tabard S, Misrahi M, Milgrom E, Schaison G: The same molecular defects of the gonadotropin-releasing hormone receptor determine a variable degree of hypogonadism in affected kindred. J Clin Endocrinol Metab 1999;84:567–572.

34 Kottler ML, Chauvin S, Lahlou N, Harris CE, Johnston CJ, Lagarde JP, Bouchard P, Farid NR, Counis R: A new compound heterozygous mutation of the gonadotropin-releasing hormone receptor (L314X, Q106R) in a woman with complete hypogonadotropic hypogonadism: Chronic estrogen administration amplifies the gonadotropin defect. J Clin Endocrinol Metab 2000;85:3002–3008.

35 Costa EM, Bedecarrats GY, Mendonca BB, Arnhold IJ, Kaiser UB, Latronico AC: Two novel mutations in the gonadotropin-releasing hormone receptor gene in Brazilian patients with hypogonadotropic hypogonadism and normal olfaction. J Clin Endocrinol Metab 2001;86:2680–2686.

36 Beranova M, Oliveira LM, Bedecarrats GY, Schipani E, Vallejo M, Ammini AC, Quintos JB, Hall JE, Martin KA, Hayes FJ, Pitteloud N, Kaiser UB, Crowley WF Jr, Seminara SB: Prevalence, phenotypic spectrum, and modes of inheritance of gonadotropin-releasing hormone receptor mutations in idiopathic hypogonadotropic hypogonadism. J Clin Endocrinol Metab 2001;86:1580–1588.

37 Maya-Nunez G, Janovick J-A, Ulloa-Aguirre A, Soderlund D, Conn PM, Mendez J-P: Molecular basis of hypogonadotropic hypogonadism: Restoration of mutant (E(90)K) GnRH receptor function by a deletion at a distant site. J Clin Endocrinol Metab 2002;87:2144–2149.

38 Silveira LFG, Stewart PM, Thomas M, Clark DA, Bouloux PMG, MacColl GS: Novel homozygous splice acceptor site GnRH receptor (GnRHR) mutation: Human GnRHR 'knockout'. J Clin Endocrinol Metab 2002;87:2973–2977.

39 Bedecarrats GY, Linher KD, Janovick JA, Beranova M, Kada F, Seminara SB, Michael-Conn P, Kaiser UB: Four naturally occurring mutations in the human GnRH receptor affect ligand binding and receptor function. Mol Cell Endocrinol 2003;205:51–64.

40 Meysing A, Kanasaki H, Bedecarrats GY, Acierno JS, Conn PM, Martin KA, Seminara SB, Hall JE, Crowley WF, Kaiser UB: GNRHR mutations in a woman with idiopathic hypogonadotropic hypogonadism highlight the differential sensitivity of luteinizing hormone and follicle-stimulating hormone to gonadotropin-releasing hormone. J Clin Endocrin Metab 2004;89:3189–3198.

41 Leanos-Miranda A, Janovick J-A, Conn PM: Receptor-misrouting: an unexpectedly prevalent and rescuable etiology in gonadotropin-releasing hormone receptor-mediated hypogonadotropic hypogonadism. J Clin Endocrinol Metab 2002;87:4825–4828.

42 Janovick J-A, Maya-Nunez G, Conn PM: Rescue of hypogonadotropic hypogonadism-causing and manufactured GnRH receptor mutants by a specific protein-folding template: Misrouted proteins as a novel disease etiology and therapeutic target. J Clin Endocrinol Metab 2002;87: 3255–3262.

43 Janovick JA, Goulet M, Bush E, Greer J, Wettlaufer DG, Conn PM: Structure-activity relations of successful pharmacologic chaperones for rescue of naturally occurring and manufactured mutants of the gonadotropin-releasing hormone receptor. J Pharmacol Exp Ther 2003;305:608–614.

44 Ulloa-Aguirre A, Janovick JA, Leanos-Miranda A, Conn PM: Misrouted cell surface GnRH receptors as a disease aetiology for congenital isolated hypogonadotrophic hypogonadism. Hum Reprod Update 2004;10:177–192.

45 Brothers SP, Cornea A, Janovick JA, Conn PM: Human loss-of-function gonadotropin-releasing hormone receptor mutants retain wild-type receptors in the endoplasmatic reticulum: Molecular basis of the dominant-negative effect. Mol Endocrinol 2004;18:1787–1797.

46 Dewailly D, Boucher A, Decanter C, Lagarde J-P, Counis R, Kottler M-L: Spontaneous pregnancy in a patient who was homozygous for the Q106R mutation in the gonadotropin-releasing hormone receptor gene. Fertil Steril 2002;77:1288–1291.

47 Pitteloud N, Boepple PA, DeCruz S, Valkenburgh SB, Crowley WF Jr, Hayes FJ: The fertile eunuch variant of idiopathic hypogonadotropic hypogonadism: Spontaneous reversal associated with a homozygous mutation in the gonadotropin-releasing hormone receptor. J Clin Endocrinol Metab 2001;86:2470–2475.
48 Söderlund D, Canto P, de la Chesnaye E, Ulloa-Aguirre A, Mendez JP: A novel homozygous mutation in the second transmembrane domain of the gonadotrophin releasing hormone receptor gene. Clin Endocrinol (Oxf) 2001;54:493–498.
49 Wolczynski S, Laudanski P, Jarzabek K, Mittre H, Lagarde JP, Kottler ML: A case of complete hypogonadotropic hypogonadism with a mutation of the gonadotropin-releasing hormone receptor gene. Steril Fertil 2003;79:442–444.
50 Seminara SB, Beranova M, Oliveira LM, Martin KA, Crowley WF, Hall JE: Successful use of pulsatile gonadotropin-releasing hormone (GnRH) for ovulation induction and pregnancy in a patient with GnRH receptor mutations. J Clin Endocrinol Metab 2000;85:556–562.
51 Layman LC, McDonough PG, Cohen DP, Maddox M, Tho SP, Reindollar RH: Familial gonadotropin-releasing hormone resistance and hypogonadotropic hypogonadism in a family with multiple affected individuals. Fertil Steril 2001;75:1148–1155.
52 Layman LC, Cohen DP, Xie J, Smith GD: Clinical phenotype and infertility treatment in a male with hypogonadotropic hypogonadism due to mutations Ala129Asp/Arg262Gln of the gonadotropin-releasing hormone receptor. Fertil Steril 2002;78:1317–1320.
53 Pitteloud N, Hayes FJ, Boepple PA, DeCruz S, Seminara SB, MacLaughlin DT, Crowley WF Jr: The role of prior pubertal development, biochemical markers of testicular maturation, and genetics in elucidating the phenotypic heterogeneity of idiopathic hypogonadotropic hypogonadism. J Clin Endocrinol Metab 2002;87:152–160.
54 Acierno JS, Shagoury JK, Bo-Abbas Y, Crowley WF, Seminara SB: A locus for autosomal-recessive idiopathic hypogonadotropic hypogonadism on chromosome 19p13.3. J Clin Endocrinol Metab 2003;88:2947–2950.
55 Genin E, Todorov AA, Clerget-Darpoux F: Optimization of genome search strategies for homozygosity mapping: Influence of marker spacing on power and threshold criteria for identification of candidate regions. Ann Hum Genet 1998;62:419–429.
56 Terasawa E, Fernandez DL: Neurobiological mechanisms of the onset of puberty in primates. Endocr Rev 2001;22:111–151.
57 Iovane A, Aumas C, de Roux N: New insights in the genetics of isolated hypogonadotropic hypogonadism. Eur J Endocrinol 2004;epub ahead of print.
58 Lee DK, Nguyen T, O'Neill GP, Cheng R, Liu Y, Howard AD, Coulombe N, Tan CP, Tang-Nguyen AT, George SR, O'Dowd BF: Discovery of a receptor related to the galanin receptors. FEBS Lett 1999;446:103–107.
59 Muir AI, Chamberlain L, Elshourbagy NA, Michalovich D, Moore DJ, Calamari A, Szekeres PG, Sarau HM, Chambers JK, Murdock P, Steplewski K, Shabon U, Miller JE, Middleton SE, Darker JG, Larminie CG, Wilson S, Bergsma DJ, Emson P, Faull R, Philpott KL, Harrison DC: AXOR12, a novel human G protein-coupled receptor, activated by the peptide KiSS-1. J Biol Chem 2001;276: 28969–28975.
60 Kotani M, Detheux M, Vandenbogaerde A, Communi D, Vanderwinden JM, Le-Poul E, Brezillon S, Tyldesley R, Suarez-Huerta N, Vandeput F, Blanpain C, Schiffmann SN, Vassart G, Parmentier M: The metastasis suppressor gene KiSS-1 encodes kisspeptins, the natural ligands of the orphan G protein-coupled receptor GPR54. J Biol Chem 2001;276:34631–34636.
61 Gottsch ML, Cunningham MJ, Smith JT, Popa SM, Acohido BV, Crowley WF, Seminara S, Clifton DK, Steiner RA: A role for kisspeptins in the regulation of gonadotropin secretion in the mouse. Endocrinology 2004;145:4073–4077.
62 Matsui H, Takatsu Y, Kumano S, Matsumoto H, Ohtaki T: Peripheral administration of metastin induces marked gonadotropin release and ovulation in the rat. Biochem Biophys Res Commun 2004;320:383–388.
63 Navarro VM, Castellano JM, Fernandez-Fernandez R, Barreiro ML, Roa J, Sanchez-Criado JE, Aguilar E, Dieguez C, Pinilla L, Tena-Sempere M: Developmental and hormonally regulated messenger ribonucleic acid expression of Kiss-1 and its putative receptor GPR54 in rat hypothalamus and potent LH releasing activity of Kiss-1 peptide. Endocrinology 2004;epub ahead of print.

64 Lee JH, Miele ME, Hicks DJ, Phillips KK, Trent JM, Weissman BE, Welch DR: KiSS-1, a novel human malignant melanoma metastasis-suppressor gene. J Natl Cancer Inst 1996;88:1731–1737.
65 Ohtaki T, Shintani Y, Honda S, Matsumoto H, Hori A, Kanehashi K, Terao Y, Kumano S, Takatsu Y, Masuda Y, Ishibashi Y, Watanabe T, Asada M, Yamada T, Suenaga M, Kitada C, Usuki S, Kurokawa T, Onda H, Nishimura O, Fujino M: Metastasis suppressor gene KiSS-1 encodes peptide ligand of a G-protein-coupled receptor. Nature 2001;411:613–617.
66 Funes S, Hedrick JA, Vassileva G, Markowitz L, Abbondanzo S, Golovko A, Yang S, Monsma FJ, Gustafson EL: The KiSS-1 receptor GPR54 is essential for the development of the murine reproductive system. Biochem Biophys Res Commun 2003;312:1357–1363.
67 Kallmann F, Schoenfeld WA, Barrera SE: The genetic aspects of primary eunuchoidism. Am J Ment Defic 1944;48:203–236.
68 de Morsier G: Etudes sur les dysraphies cranio-encephaliques. I. Agenesie des lobes olfactifs (telencephaloschizis lateral) et des commissures calleuse et anterieure (telencephaloschizis median). La dysplasie olfacto genitale. Schweiz Arch Neurol Neurochir Psychiatr 1954;74:309–361.
69 Rugarli EI: Kallmann syndrome and the link between olfactory and reproductive development. Am J Hum Genet 1999;65:943–948.
70 Hardelin JP, Levilliers J, del-Castillo I, Cohen-Salmon M, Legouis R, Blanchard S, Compain S, Bouloux P, Kirk J, Moraine C, et al.: X chromosome-linked Kallmann syndrome: Stop mutations validate the candidate gene. Proc Natl Acad Sci USA 1992;89:8190–8194.
71 Maya-Nunez G, Zenteno JC, Ulloa-Aguirre A, Kofman-Alfaro S, Mendez JP: A recurrent missense mutation in the KAL gene in patients with X-linked Kallmann's syndrome. J Clin Endocrinol Metab 1998;83:1650–1653.
72 Soderlund D, Canto P, Mendez JP: Identification of three novel mutations in the KAL1 gene in patients with Kallmann syndrome. J Clin Endocrinol Metab 2002;87:2589–2592.
73 Massin N, Pecheux C, Eloit C, Bensimon JL, Galey J, Kuttenn F, Hardelin JP, Dode C, Touraine P: X chromosome-linked Kallmann syndrome: Clinical heterogeneity in three siblings carrying an intragenic deletion of the KAL-1 gene. J Clin Endocrinol Metab 2003;88:2003–2008.
74 Hu Y, Tanriverdi F, MacColl GS, Bouloux PM: Kallmann's syndrome: Molecular pathogenesis. Int J Biochem Cell Biol 2003;35:1157–1162.
75 Soussi-Yanicostas N, de-Castro F, Julliard AK, Perfettini I, Chedotal A, Petit C: Anosmin-1, defective in the X-linked form of Kallmann syndrome, promotes axonal branch formation from olfactory bulb output neurons. Cell 2002;109:217–228.
76 MacColl G, Bouloux P, Quinton R: Kallmann syndrome: Adhesion, afferents, and anosmia. Neuron 2002;34:675–678.
77 Izumi Y, Tatsumi K, Okamoto S, Ogawa T, Hosokawa A, Matsuo T, Kato Y, Fukui H, Amino N: Analysis of the KAL1 gene in 19 Japanese patients with Kallmann syndrome. Endocr J 2001;48: 143–149.
78 Oliveira LM, Seminara SB, Beranova M, Hayes FJ, Valkenburgh SB, Schipani E, Costa EM, Latronico AC, Crowley WF Jr, Vallejo M: The importance of autosomal genes in Kallmann syndrome: Genotype-phenotype correlations and neuroendocrine characteristics. J Clin Endocrinol Metab 2001;86:1532–1538.
79 Quinton R, Duke VM, Robertson A, Kirk JM, Matfin G, de-Zoysa PA, Azcona C, MacColl GS, Jacobs HS, Conway GS, Besser M, Stanhope RG, Bouloux PM: Idiopathic gonadotrophin deficiency: Genetic questions addressed through phenotypic characterization. Clin Endocrinol (Oxf) 2001;55:163–174.
80 Yazaki N, Hosoi Y, Kawabata K, Miyake A, Minami M, Satoh M, Ohta M, Kawasaki T, Itoh N: Differential expression patterns of mRNAs for members of the fibroblast growth factor receptor family, FGFR-1-FGFR-4, in rat brain. J Neurosci Res 1994;37:445–452.
81 Hebert JM, Lin M, Partanen J, Rossant J, McConnell SK: FGF signaling through FGFR1 is required for olfactory bulb morphogenesis. Development 2003;130:1101–1111.

Nicolas de Roux, MD, PhD, INSERM U584, Hormone Targets
Medical Faculty, Necker-Enfants Malades, 156, rue de Vaugirard, FR–75015 Paris (France)
Tel. +33 1 40615309, Fax +33 1 43060443, E-Mail deroux@necker.fr

Delemarre-van de Waal HA (ed): Abnormalities in Puberty. Scientific and Clinical Advances.
Endocr Dev. Basel, Karger, 2005, vol 8, pp 81–93

Hypothalamic Hamartoma: A Paradigm/Model for Studying the Onset of Puberty

Heike Jung, Anne-Simone Parent, Sergio R. Ojeda

Division of Neuroscience, Oregon National Primate Research Center/Oregon Health & Science University, Beaverton, Oreg., USA

Abstract

This article discusses the potential mechanisms by which hypothalamic hamartomas (HHs) are formed and cause precocious puberty. The hypothesis is presented suggesting that HHs accelerate sexual development by producing bioactive substances that mimic – in an accelerated time-course – the cascade of events underlying the normal initiation of puberty. It is also proposed that because HHs contain key transcriptional and signaling networks required to initiate and sustain a pubertal mode of gonadotropin-releasing hormone (GnRH) release, they are able to trigger the pubertal process at an earlier age. The cellular components of this activating complex may include: (a) neurons able to produce GnRH within the HH: (b) controlling neurons synaptically connected to GnRH neurons in the HH itself and/or to neuronal networks (including GnRH neurons) in the patient's hypothalamus, and (c) signaling-competent astrocytic and ependymoglial cells. It is also possible that the developmental abnormalities leading to the formation of HHs result from sporadic defects affecting the same genes and hence the same morphogenic pathways involved in the embryonic development of the ventral hypothalamus and the floor of the third ventricle.

Hamartomas of the central nervous system are rare congenital non-neoplastic lesions containing mature tissue in a heterotopic location; hamartomas are almost exclusively located at the base of the hypothalamus where they develop as an outgrowth of the floor of the third ventricle [1–3]. In most cases, hypothalamic hamartomas (HHs) contain neurons and astroglial cells of normal aspect [3, 4], in addition to ependymoglial-like cells that may be scattered throughout the mass of tissue or arranged in clusters [5]. Neuronal processes reaching adjacent structures frequently form bundles of myelinated fibers [1]. Overall, both neurons and glial cells appear to be normal, although in several instances the number of astrocytes seems to be increased, and some of them may show features typical of reactive astrocytes [1, 2, 5].

Most symptomatic HHs are associated with central precocious puberty [2] and/or gelastic seizures, a form of ictal laughter [6–9]. In fact, a literature review describing 50 cases of hamartomas over a time period of 47 years (1934–1981), demonstrated that only 11 of them – diagnosed at autopsy – were asymptomatic [1]. Neither the factors underlying the formation of HHs nor the mechanism(s) by which HHs trigger the pubertal process and/or cause gelastic seizures have been identified. Although it is clear that HHs represent a developmental aberration, their presence has not been specifically associated to any genetic disorder; accordingly, HHs are classified as congenital malformations of the hypothalamus without familiar recurrence [10]. It is, however, interesting to note that HHs can be detected in a number of pleiotropic disorders of human development [3, 11]. Despite this prevalence, only in Pallister-Hall syndrome (PHS) the presence of HH is a constant feature with diagnostic value [12]. Though intriguing, this feature does not explain why the hamartoma mass is the only malformation detected in the large majority of HH cases thus far reported. In contrast, HHs in PHS are always detected in association with a plethora of other abnormalities including central polydactyly, pituitary hypoplasia, dysplastic nails, imperforated anus, and bifid epiglottis [11, 13].

Sexual precocity caused by a HH occurs at a much earlier age than in idiopathic precocious puberty of central origin [14]. The mechanisms by which HHs causes early onset of the pubertal process remain unknown. Mechanical pressure, autonomous gonadotropin-releasing hormone (GnRH) secretion, transsynaptic activation via myelinated fibers connecting the hamartoma to the hypothalamus, and secretion of glial products able to stimulate the patient's GnRH neuronal network are the most favored mechanisms invoked [reviewed in 1, 3, 15]. The finding that some HH do not induce sexual precocity – despite a hypothalamic location similar to that of HH associated with precocious puberty [16, 17] – argues against the idea of mechanical factors underlying HH-induced precocious puberty. Instead, it strengthens the concept that HHs accelerate sexual development because they produce substances capable of eliciting gonadotropin secretion prematurely, either directly or indirectly, via stimulation of GnRH production. If one accepts the general validity of this concept, HHs can be envisioned as the keepers of crucial information that can help us in identifying those factors that, operating within the normal hypothalamus, set in motion the pubertal process.

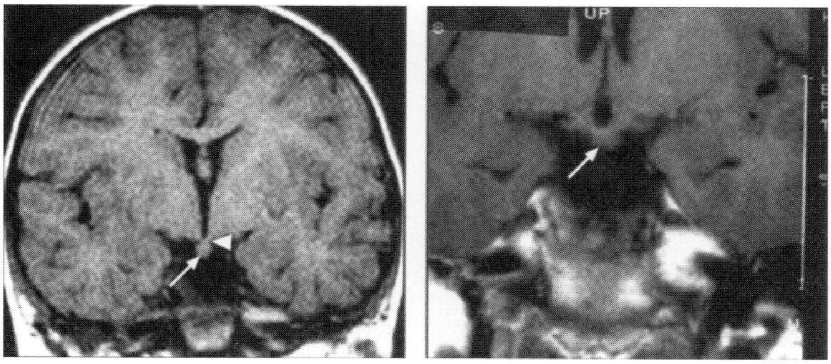

a b

Fig. 1. ***a*** Coronal MRI of the brain showing a small hypothalamic mass (arrow), diagnosed as a parahypothalamic hamartoma suspended from a peduncle (arrowhead), and associated with isolated precocious puberty. ***b*** Coronal MRI view of the brain of another patient showing a hamartoma (arrow) broadly attached to the hypothalamus in a parahypothalamic position. This hamartoma also induced isolated sexual precocity.

Anatomical Aspects

Hypothalamic hamartomas are either located adjacent to hypothalamic structures – in a parahypothalamic position – or infiltrating the hypothalamus [7, 18]. Some parahypothalamic hamartomas are attached to the hypothalamus by a peduncle (fig. 1a), while others are broadly attached (fig. 1b) to the base of the third ventricle [18]. In a series of 34 patients with HH, 12 exhibited seizures – either isolated or in combination with sexual precocity. In almost all of them (11 of 12) the HH had infiltrated the hypothalamus (fig. 2a, b) [17]. The use of advanced imaging techniques, such as magnetic resonance proton spectroscopy, indicated that a large portion of HHs associated with seizure activity infiltrate the hypothalamus predominantly between the fornix, the mamillary body and the mammillothalamic tract, tending to displace the post-commissural fornix and hypothalamic gray matter anterolaterally [19]. In the same series of patients, larger HHs were shown to be associated with both sexual precocity and epileptic disorder [19], supporting the observation that HHs of a diameter above 10 mm are more likely associated with seizure activity either isolated or in combination with precocious puberty [7, 17]. The association of some of these large HHs with precocious puberty may not, however, be related at all to their size, but instead to the infiltration of ventral hypothalamic regions involved in the control of GnRH secretion. In contrast to HH associated with epilepsy, those associated with sexual precocity are frequently pedunculated [17, 18]. Yet, little is known about the chemical nature

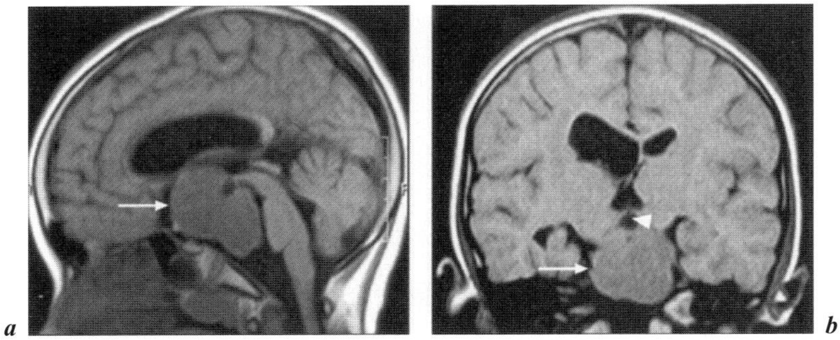

Fig. 2. ***a*** Sagittal MRI view revealing a large, broad-based intrahypothalamic hamartoma (arrow). The hamartoma induced sexual precocity combined with epileptic seizures. ***b*** Dorsal MRI section of the same patient showing infiltration of the hypothalamus and the third ventricle (arrowhead) by the large hamartoma (arrow).

of the structural connections and/or cell-cell signaling pathways linking the hamartoma tissue with surrounding hypothalamic structures.

An interesting aspect of HHs is the existence of an apparent relationship between their anatomical position in the hypothalamus and the sex of the patient. In a series of 34 patients with HH associated with sexual precocity and/or gelastic seizure activity, a parahypothalamic, pedunculated, location of these malformations was seen predominantly in girls and was more frequently associated with isolated precocious puberty [17]. In contrast, male patients appeared to be at a higher risk of developing intrahypothalamic HHs compromising the third ventricle. These differences may reflect the establishment of gender-specific structural connections within the hypothalamus itself and/or with the HH. Since the first description of sex-related differences in neuronal connectivity within the developing hypothalamus [20] many more examples of sex-specific organization of hypothalamic nuclei have been described [for review, see 21]. Although cell number, size and density tended to be larger in males in the majority of sexually dimorphic areas of the hypothalamus, in some regions sexual dimorphism favors females. Sex differences in glial morphology have also been described in the arcuate nucleus of the neonate rat [22]. However, neither the orientation nor the density of glia seems to contribute to a more intense medial to lateral migration of neurons in the preoptic area of male rats [23], suggesting that the differences in migration are due to other influences, such as a direct effect of sex steroids on the migrating neurons. A factor that might play a role in brain sexual differentiation is the existence of developmental programs determined, not by gonadal steroids, but instead by the complement of sex chromosome genes expressed in phenotypically diverse neural cell populations [24]. Whether gonadal steroids and/or sex chromosome genes influence the location of HHs and/or their integration to surrounding structures in the developing human hypothalamus remains to be determined. Nonetheless, there is little doubt that gender is an important factor influencing the frequency of pubertal manifestations in patients with HH (more evident in girls than boys) [14, 17, 18, 25], a feature consistent with the overall higher incidence of idiopathic sexual precocity in females than males [10].

Potential Mechanisms Underlying Sexual Precocity Induced by HHs

Although a variety of organic lesions – including tumors, cranial irradiation, infection, hydrocephalus or trauma – can induce sexual precocity [26], the diverse nature of these lesions suggests that they accelerate the pubertal process, not by producing bioactive substances, but instead via nonspecific activation of the surrounding hypothalamic tissue. As in the case of HHs, however, this activation occurs only if the lesion affects areas of the hypothalamus near to, or implicated in the control of, the GnRH neuronal network.

In contrast to organic lesions, HHs with similar locations [see for instance 17] can either induce precocious puberty, epileptic seizures, or both, suggesting that – as indicated above – it is the nature of their connectivity and/or secretory capacity that determine their ability to hasten sexual development.

Because HHs are composed of normal – but ectopically situated – neural elements, including neurons, glial cells and their processes, it would appear reasonable to argue that HHs represent a focal site of autonomous neuroendocrine activity able to initiate and sustain the pubertal process using mechanisms similar to those that – initiated within the hypothalamus – underlie the normal initiation of puberty (fig. 3). Support for this concept comes from the detection of GnRH neurons within some HHs [27], a finding that led to the hypothesis that these neurons represent a functionally independent cohort of neurosecretory cells able to prematurely activate endogenous pulsatile GnRH release and induce premature sexual maturation [27, 28] (fig. 3). However, not all HHs associated with sexual precocity contain GnRH neurons [29–31]. We recently reported [31] two cases of sexual precocity caused by HHs in which the malformation, instead of containing GnRH neurons, displayed a network of astrocytes expressing transforming growth factor-α (TGFα) and its erbB-1 receptor. TGFα is a growth factor member of the epidermal growth factor family, involved in mediating the facilitatory control that glial cells exert on the GnRH neuronal network [32]. According to these and other results obtained in laboratory animals [reviewed in 32, 33], it has been proposed that HHs containing

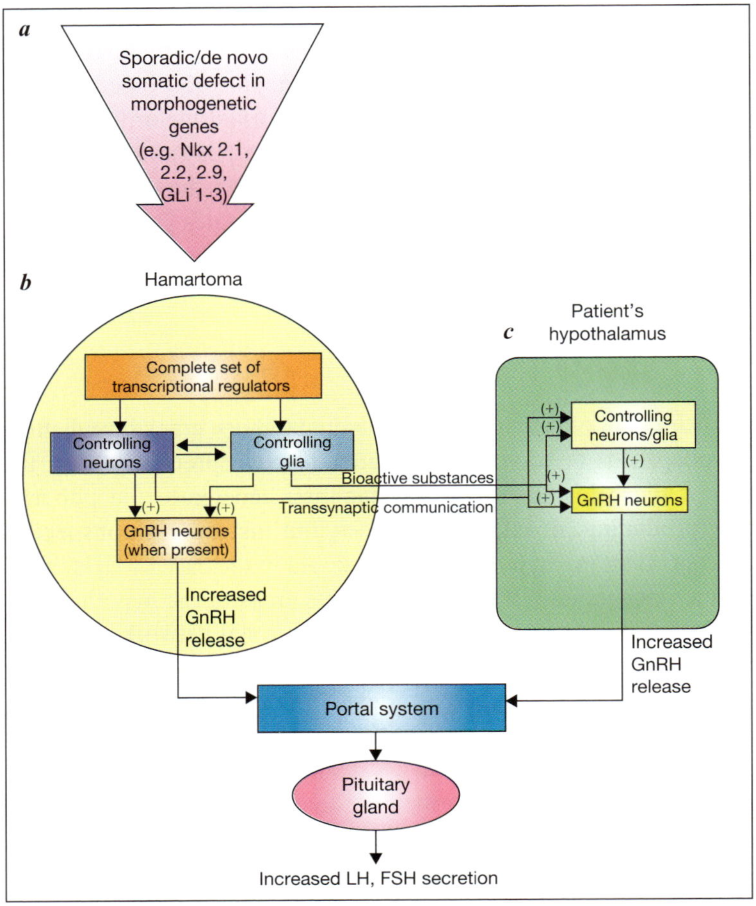

Fig. 3. Potential mechanisms implicated in the development of HHs, and underlying the ability of HHs to activate GnRH secretion and induce sexual precocity. ***a*** The formation of an HH may be determined by sporadic/de novo somatic mutations in genes required for hypothalamic morphogenesis. The identity of genes whose defects lead to formation of HHs is not known. ***b*** The HH itself may contain all the necessary components to activate GnRH release either from GnRH neurons intrinsic to the HH or those of the patient's hypothalamus. ***c*** The patient's hypothalamus can respond to both bioactive substances produced by the HH and to transsynaptic inputs provided by neuronal connections established between the HH and the hypothalamus.

TGFα-producing cells secrete bioactive substances able to act on GnRH neurons located on adjacent, normal hypothalamic tissue to stimulate GnRH secretion [15, 31] (fig. 3). In keeping with this notion, cells genetically engineered to produce TGFα were found to induce sexual maturation in female rats when grafted near either GnRH nerve terminals or GnRH cell bodies [34]. A very recent study [35] showed that normal ependymoglial cells (which, as indicated above, are also present in HHs) contain erbB-1 receptors and respond to TGFα with production of prostaglandin E_2 (PGE_2) and transforming growth factor-β1, two molecules involved in the control of GnRH neuronal function. While PGE_2 stimulates GnRH release in vivo [36] and in vitro [37], TGFβ1 appears to only stimulate GnRH release from a GnRH neuronal cell line [38]. However, TGFβ1 increases expression of the GnRH gene in both this GnRH-secreting cell line [38] and native GnRH neurons in situ [39]. Thus, the presence of astrocytes and ependymoglial cells in HHs, coupled to the expression of both TGFα and its receptor, indicate that HHs have the necessary components to engage in the same signaling events that, set in motion by erbB-1 signaling in normal hypothalamic astrocytes and ependymoglial cells of the median eminence, lead to stimulation of GnRH secretion at puberty [40].

Disruption of a melatonin-mediated inhibitory control of the GnRH secreting system has been also suggested as another potential mechanism by which HH may accelerate sexual development [41, 42]. However, others have questioned this idea and have instead favored the concept proposed above, i.e. that malformations and/or tumors compromising the pineal gland induce central precocious puberty because they produce bioactive substances [43]. In fact, HHs have been found to produce several neuropeptides in addition to GnRH and TGFα, including corticotrophin-releasing hormone (CRH) [7, 44], met-enkephalin [7], growth hormone [45], β-endorphin and oxytocin [46], and somatostatin and thyroid-stimulating hormone [47]. Importantly, some of these peptides have been shown to be involved in the regulation of GnRH secretion [48–52].

These considerations bring up the issue of the potential mechanisms underlying the development of HHs. It would appear intuitively logical to assume that HHs develop as a consequence of discrete defects of the same processes governing normal embryonic hypothalamic development (fig. 3). Initial support for this idea comes from the identification in PHS patients [53] of mutations in the Gli3 gene, a regulator of the sonic hedgehog protein (SHH) morphogenic pathway [54, 55]. SHH controls hypothalamic development, at least in part, by promoting the transcriptional activity of three genes of the Nkx family of homeodomain genes: T/ebp/Nkx2.1, Nkx 2.2 and Nkx 2.9 [56]. T/ebp also known as TTF-1 is required for the development of several hypothalamic nuclei, including the ventromedial and arcuate nucleus [57]. Importantly, T/ebp null mice fail to form the ventral portion of the third ventricle [57], indicating that T/ebp plays a critical role in the morphogenesis of the very same region implicated in the formation of HHs. Nkx 2.2, on the other hand, plays a critical role in specifying ventral neuronal identities in response to inductive SHH signaling [58]. Nkx 2.9 expression in the ventral nervous system precedes and spatially overlaps that of Nkx 2.2 [59], suggesting a close functional relationship among the two.

Though important in PHS, it does not appear that mutations of the Gli3 gene are responsible for the development of HHs. Mice carrying targeted mutations of the same region in the Gli3 gene identified in patients with PHS do not develop HHs despite exhibiting most of the abnormalities present in PHS [60]. While this finding might simply reflect a lack of involvement of Gli3 mutations in the genesis of HH, it is important to note that mutations of the Gli3 gene display marked phenotypic heterogeneity [60], showing either gain or loss-of function in their ability to inhibit SHH signaling [54, 55]. It is, therefore, possible that low-penetrance mutations of this and/or other downstream genes involved in hypothalamic morphogenesis might lead to the isolated formation of HHs. In recent studies, we have observed that expression of T/ebp in a glial progenitor cell line prevents the proliferative response of the cells to TGFα stimulation [61], and promotes the differentiation of the cells towards a tanycytic, ependymoglial phenotype. Thus, it is possible that defects in morphogenetic pathways controlling development of the ventral hypothalamus might result in abnormalities favoring the formation of HHs (fig. 3). A complicating feature of this interpretation is the almost unavoidable need to invoke the existence of cell-specific abnormalities affecting discrete cellular subsets of the embryonic hypothalamus. These cellular subsets would also have to be embryologically linked to originate normal sub-domains of the hypothalamic landscape. A precedent for such cell-specific genetic abnormality can be found in the sporadic appearance of mutations in *UBE3A*, the imprinted gene affected in Angelman syndrome [62]. The UBE3A gene, which encodes a ubiquitin ligase, is expressed biparentally in all cells except for Purkinje, hippocampal and olfactory mitral neurons [62], in which only the maternal allele is expressed. In these cells, the paternal allele is silenced, i.e. the gene is maternally imprinted. Mutations of the expressed maternal allele lead to the neurological symptoms characteristic of Angelman syndrome, including ataxia, tremor, epilepsy and learning deficits.

Three imprinted genes with paternal monoallelic expression, *Peg3*, *Mest/Peg1* and *Necdin,* are expressed in the developing hypothalamus [63–65]. Importantly, mice carrying mutations in the *Mest/Peg1* and *Necdin* genes do not exhibit gross abnormalities of hypothalamic structure, but instead they display defects in hypothalamic-dependent behaviors [64], and discrete defects in the differentiation/survival of specific hypothalamic cell populations, including oxytocin and GnRH neurons [65]. Necdin is one of the paternally imprinted genes involved in Prader-Willy syndrome [66]; Necdin-deficient mice show some hypothalamic and behavioral abnormalities similar to those seen in patients affected by Prader-Willi syndrome [65]. It would not be unreasonable, therefore, to entertain the almost heretical possibility that formation of HHs involves the loss of expression of imprinted genes in 'uniparental' cells of the hypothalamus [67, 68]. In support of this idea, recent studies in the mouse have made it abundantly clear that imprinted genes play a crucial role in brain development [68, 69]. Obviously, new strategies will have to be developed to clarify this important issue.

Using Affymetrix arrays, we recently interrogated 18,400 genes to compare a HH associated with precocious puberty with HHs that do not induce sexual precocity and found a discrete subset of genes whose expression is significantly changed in the HH associated with sexual precocity in comparison to the other HHs [Parent et al., unpubl. results]. It is possible that an in-depth analysis of these results will provide us with valuable hints towards the identification of the gene networks that operating within HHs might be responsible for their puberty-inducing activity.

Conclusion

Based on the above considerations, we hypothesize that hypothalamic hamartomas (HHs) accelerate sexual development by producing bioactive substances that mimic – in a highly compressed time frame – the cascade of events underlying the normal initiation of puberty. We also submit that, because HHs are congenital malformations and contain the key transcriptional and signaling networks required to initiate and sustain a pubertal mode of GnRH release, they are able to trigger the pubertal process at a much earlier age than other forms of precocious puberty, including idiopathic puberty of central origin. The cellular components of this activating complex may include neurons able to produce GnRH, controlling neuronal networks synaptically connected to GnRH neurons in the HH itself and/or to neurons (including GnRH neurons) in the patient's hypothalamus, in addition to astrocytes and ependymoglial cells endowed with glia-to-neuron signaling capabilities. Lastly, it is also possible that the developmental abnormalities leading to the formation of HHs result from sporadic/de novo defects affecting the same homeotic genes and hence the same pathways involved in the embryonic development of the ventral hypothalamus and the floor of the third ventricle. The possibility that some of these genes are imprinted and expressed in 'uniparental' cells should also been given proper consideration. It thus appears that the functional and molecular analysis of HHs may offer new and compelling insights into both the etiology of sexual precocity and the central mechanisms underlying the initiation of normal puberty.

Acknowledgments

This research was supported by NIH grants HD-25123, MH-065438, NICHD/NIH through cooperative U54 HD18185 as part of the Specialized Cooperative Centers Program in Reproduction Research, and RR00163 for the operation of the Oregon National Primate Research Center. ASP was a postdoctoral research fellow supported by the FNRS (Fonds National de la Recherche Scientifique, Belgium) and MH-065438.

References

1 Zuniga OF, Tanner SM, Wild WO, Mosier HD Jr: Hamartoma of CNS associated with precocious puberty. Am J Dis Child 1983;137:127–133.
2 Richter RB: True hamartoma of the hypothalamus associated with pubertas praecox. J Neuropathol Exp Neurol 1951;10:368–383.
3 Freeman JL: The anatomy and embryology of the hypothalamus in relation to hypothalamic hamartomas. Epileptic Disord 2003;5:177–186.
4 Burger PC, Scheithauer BW, Vogel FS: Surgical Pathology of the Nervous System and Its Coverings. New York, Churchill-Livingstone, 1991.
5 Bedwell SF, Lindenberg R: A hypothalamic hamartoma with dendritic proliferation and other neuronal changes associated with 'blastomatoid' reaction of astrocytes. J Neuropathol Exp Neurol 1961;20:219–236.
6 Dammann O, Commentz JC, Valdueza JM, Christante L, Bentele KH: Gelastic epilepsy and precocious puberty in hamartoma of the hypothalamus. Klin Paediatr 1991;203:439–447.
7 Valdueza JM, Cristante L, Dammann O, Bentele K, Vortmeyer A, Saeger W, Padberg B, Freitag J, Herrmann H-D: Hypothalamic hamartomas: With special reference to gelastic epilepsy and surgery. Neurosurgery 1994;34:949–958.
8 Arroyo S, Santamaría J, Sanmartí F, Lomeña F, Catafau A, Casamitjana R, Setoain J, Tolosa E: Ictal laughter associated with paroxysmal hypothalamopituitary dysfunction. Epilepsia 1997;38: 114–117.
9 Breningstall GN: Gelastic seizures, precocious puberty, and hypothalamic hamartoma. Neurology 2004;35:1180–1183.
10 Grumbach MM, Styne DM: Puberty: Ontogeny, neuroendocrinology, physiology, and disorders; in Larsen PR, Kronenberg HM, Melmed S, Polonsky KS (eds): Williams Textbook of Endocrinology, ed 10. Philadelphia, Saunders, 2003, pp 1115–1286.
11 Killoran CE, Abbott M, McKusick VA, Biesecker LG: Overlap of PIV syndrome, VACTERL and Pallister-Hall syndrome: Clinical and molecular analysis. Clin Genet 2000;58:28–30.
12 Biesecker LG, Abbott M, Allen J, Clericuzio C, Feuillan P, Graham JM Jr, Hall J, Kang S, Olney AH, Lefton D, Neri G, Peters K, Verloes A: Report from the workshop on Pallister-Hall syndrome and related phenotypes. Am J Med Genet 1996;65:76–81.
13 Biesecker LG, Graham JM: Pallister-Hall syndrome. J Med Genet 1996;33:585–589.
14 Hibi I, Fujiwara K: Precocious puberty of cerebral origin: A cooperative study in Japan. Prog Exp Tumor Res 1987;30:224–238.
15 Jung H, Ojeda SR: Pathogenesis of precocious puberty in hypothalamic harmartoma. Horm Res 2002;57(suppl 2):31–34.
16 Sato M, Ushio Y, Arita N, Mogami H: Hypothalamic hamartoma: Report of two cases. Neurosurgery 1985;16:198–206.
17 Jung H, Probst EN, Hauffa BP, Partsch C-J, Dammann O: Association of morphological characteristics with precocious puberty and/or gelastic seizures in hypothalamic hamartoma. J Clin Endocrinol Metab 2003;88:4590–4595.
18 Debeneix C, Bourgeois M, Trivin C, Sainte-Rose C, Brauner R: Hypothalamic hamartoma: Comparison of clinical presentation and magnetic resonance images. Horm Res 2001;56:12–18.

19 Freeman JL, Coleman LT, Wellard RM, Kean MJ, Rosenfield JV, Jackson GD, Berkovic SF, Harvey AS: MR imaging and spectroscopic study of epileptogenic hypothalamic hamartomas: Analysis of 72 cases. Am J Neuroradiol 2004;25:450–462.
20 Raisman G, Field PM: Sexual dimorphism in the preoptic area of the rat. Science 1971;173: 731–733.
21 Simerly RB: Wired for reproduction: Organization and development of sexually dimorphic circuits in the mammalian forebrain. Annu Rev Neurosci 2002;25:507–536.
22 Mong JA, Glaser E, McCarthy MM: Gonadal steroids promote glial differentiation and alter neuronal morphology in the developing hypothalamus in a regionally specific manner. J Neurosci 1999;19:1464–1472.
23 Henderson RG, Brown AE, Tobet SA: Sex differences in cell migration in the preoptic area/ anterior hypothalamus of mice. Neurobiology 1999;41:252–266.
24 Carruth LL, Reisert I, Arnold AP: Sex chromosome genes directly affect brain sexual differentiation. Nat Neurosci 2002;5:933–934.
25 Arita K, Ikawa F, Kurisu K, Sumida M, Harada K, Uozumi T, Monden S, Yoshida J, Nishi Y: The relationship between magnetic resonance imaging findings and clinical manifestations of hypothalamic hamartoma. J Neurosurg 1999;91:212–220.
26 Grumbach MM, Kaplan SL: Recent advances in the diagnosis and management of sexual precocity. Acta Paediatr Jpn 1988;30:155–175.
27 Judge DM, Kulin HE, Page R, Santen R, Trapukda S: Hypothalamic hamartoma: A source of luteinizing-hormone-releasing factor in precocious puberty. N Engl J Med 1977;296:7–10.
28 Mahachoklertwattana P, Kaplan SL, Grumbach MM: The luteinizing hormone-releasing hormone-secreting hypothalamic hamartoma is a congenital malformation: Natural history. Clin Endocrinol Metab 1993;77:118–124.
29 Markin RS, Leibrock LG, Huseman CA, McComb RD: Hypothalamic hamartoma: A report of 2 cases. Pediatr Neurosci 1987;13:19–26.
30 Kammer KS, Perlman K, Humphreys RP, Howard NJ: Clinical and surgical aspects of hypothalamic hamartoma associated with precocious puberty in a 15-month-old boy. Child's Brain 1980;6:150–157.
31 Jung H, Carmel P, Schwartz MS, Witkin JW, Bentele KHP, Westphal M, Piatt JH, Costa ME, Cornea A, Ma YJ, Ojeda SR: Some hypothalamic hamartomas contain transforming growth factor alpha, a puberty-inducing growth factor, but not luteinizing hormone-releasing hormone neurons. J Clin Endocrinol Metab 1999;84:4695–4701.
32 Ojeda SR, Prevot V, Heger S, Lomniczi A, Dziedzic B, Mungenast A: Glia-to-neuron signaling and the neuroendocrine control of female puberty. Ann Med 2003;35:244–255.
33 Ojeda SR, Ma YJ: The role of growth factors in the neuroendocrine control of female sexual development. Curr Opin Endocrinol Diab 1995;2:148–156.
34 Rage F, Hill DF, Sena-Esteves M, Breakefield XO, Coffey RJ, Costa ME, McCann SM, Ojeda SR: Targeting transforming growth factor-α expression to discrete loci of the neuroendocrine brain induces female sexual precocity. Proc Natl Acad Sci USA 1997;94:2735–2740.
35 Prevot V, Cornea A, Mungenast A, Smiley G, Ojeda SR: Activation of erbB-1 signaling in tanycytes of the median eminence stimulates transforming growth factor-β_1 release via prostaglandin E2 production and induces cell plasticity. J Neurosci 2003;23:10622–10632.
36 Ojeda SR, Negro-Vilar A, McCann SM: Release of prostaglandin E (PGEs) by hypothalamic tissue: Evidence for their involvement in catecholamine-induced LHRH release. Endocrinology 1979;104:617–624.
37 Ma YJ, Berg-von der Emde K, Rage F, Wetsel WC, Ojeda SR: Hypothalamic astrocytes respond to transforming growth factor alpha with secretion of neuroactive substances that stimulate the release of luteinizing hormone-releasing hormone. Endocrinology 1997;138:19–25.
38 Galbiati M, Zanisi M, Messi E, Cavarretta I, Martini L, Melcangi RC: Transforming growth factor-β and astrocytic conditioned medium influence luteinizing hormone-releasing hormone gene expression in the hypothalamic cell line GT1. Endocrinology 1996;137:5605–5609.
39 Bouret S, De Seranno S, Beauvillain JC, Prevot V: Transforming growth factor β_1 may directly influence gonadotropin-releasing hormone gene expression in the rat hypothalamus. Endocrinology 2004;145:1794–1801.

40 Ojeda SR, Terasawa E: Neuroendocrine regulation of puberty; in Pfaff D, Arnold A, Etgen A, Fahrbach S, Moss R, Rubin R (eds): Hormones, Brain and Behavior. New York, Elsevier, 2002, vol 4, pp 589–659.
41 Commentz JC, Helmke K: Precocious puberty and decreased melatonin secretion due to a hypothalamic hamartoma. Horm Res 1995;44:271–275.
42 Commentz JC, Uhlig H, Henke A, Hellwege HH, Willig RP: Melatonin and 6-hydroxymelatonin sulfate excretion is inversely correlated with gonadal development in children. Horm Res 1997;47:97–101.
43 Rivarola M, Belgorosky A, Mendilaharzu H, Vidal G: Precocious puberty in children with tumours of the suprasellar and pineal areas: Organic central precocious puberty. Acta Paediatr 2001;90:751–756.
44 Voyadzis JM, Guttman-Bauman I, Santi M, Cogen P: Hypothalamic hamartoma secreting corticotropin-releasing hormone. Case report. J Neurosurg 2004;100(2 suppl):212–216.
45 Asa SL, Bilbao JM, Kovacs K, Linfoot JA: Hypothalamic neuronal hamartoma associated with pituitary growth hormone cell adenoma and acromegaly. Acta Neuropathol (Berl) 1980;52: 231–234.
46 Nishio S, Fujiwara S, Aiko Y, Takeshita I, Fukui M: Hypothalamic hamartoma. Report of two cases. J Neurosurg 1989;70:640–645.
47 Hochman HI, Judge DM, Reichlin S: Precocious puberty and hypothalamic hamartoma. Pediatrics 1981;67:236–244.
48 Rivest S, Rivier C: The role of corticotropin-releasing factor and interleukin-1 in the regulation of neurons controlling reproductive functions. Endocr Rev 1995;16:177–199.
49 Selvage D, Johnston CA: Central stimulatory influence of oxytocin on preovulatory gonadotropin-releasing hormone requires more than the median eminence. Neuroendocrinology 2001;74: 129–134.
50 Tellam DJ, Mohammad YN, Lovejoy DA: Molecular integration of hypothalamo-pituitary-adrenal axis-related neurohormones on the GnRH neuron. Biochem Cell Biol 2000;78:205–216.
51 Van Vugt HH, Swarts JJM, Van De Heijning BJM, Van De Beek EM: Centrally applied somatostatin inhibits the luteinizing hormone surge in female rats. Soc Neurosci Abstr 2003;abstr 237.5.
52 Wilson ME: The impact of the GH-IGF-I axis on gonadotropin secretion: Inferences from animal models. J Pediatr Endocrinol Metab 2001;14:115–140.
53 Kang S, Graham JM Jr, Olney AH, Biesecker LG: GLI3 frameshift mutations cause autosomal dominant Pallister-Hall syndrome. Nat Genet 1997;15:266–268.
54 Michaud JL: The developmental program of the hypothalamus and its disorders. Clin Genet 2001;60:255–263.
55 Villavicencio EH, Walterhouse DO, Iannaccone PM: The sonic hedgehog-patched-glial pathway in human development and disease. Am J Hum Genet 2000;67:1047–1054.
56 Pabst O, Herbrand H, Takuma N, Arnold HH: NKX2 gene expression in neuroectoderm but not in mesendodermally derived structures depends on sonic hedgehog in mouse embryos. Dev Genes Evol 2000;210:47–50.
57 Kimura S, Hara Y, Pineau T, Fernandez-Salguero P, Fox CH, Ward JM, Gonzalez FJ: The *T/ebp* null mouse: Thyroid-specific enhancer-binding protein is essential for the organogenesis of the thyroid, lung, ventral forebrain, and pituitary. Genes Dev 1996;10:60–69.
58 Briscoe J, Sussel L, Serup P, Hartigan-O'Connor DJ, Jessell TM, Rubenstein JLR, Ericson J: Homeobox gene *Nkx*2.2 and specification of neuronal identity by graded sonic hedgehog signalling. Nature 1999;398:622–626.
59 Pabst O, Herbrand H, Arnold H-H: Nkx2–9 is a novel homeobox transcription factor which demarcates ventral domains in the developing mouse CNS. Mech Dev 1998;73:85–93.
60 Böse J, Grotewold L, Rüther U: Pallister-Hall syndrome phenotype in mice mutant for *Gli3*. Hum Mol Genet 2002;11:1129–1135.
61 Lomniczi A, Smiley G, Mastronardi C, Cho GJ, Damante G, Hill DF, Jeong JK, Lee BJ, Ojeda SR: TTF-1, a homeodomain protein required for diencephalic morphogenesis, induces the differentiation of specialized hypothalamic glial cells (abstract/viewer). Washington, Society for Neuroscience, 2004, program 758.2.
62 Jiang Y-H, Lev-Lehman E, Bressler J, Tsai T-F, Beaudet AL: Genetics of Angelman syndrome. Am J Hum Genet 1999;65:1–6.

63 Kuroiwa Y, Kaneko-Ishino T, Kagitani F, Kohda T, Li LL, Tada M, Suzuki R, Yokoyama M, Shiroishi T, Wakana S, Barton SC, Ishino F, Surani MA: Peg3 imprinted gene on proximal chromosome 7 encodes for a zinc finger protein. Nat Genet 1996;12:186–190.
64 Lefebvre L, Viville S, Barton SC, Ishino F, Keverne EB, Surani MA: Abnormal maternal behaviour and growth retardation associated with loss of the imprinted gene *Mest*. Nat Genet 1998;20:163–169.
65 Muscatelli F, Abrous DN, Massacier A, Boccaccio I, Le Moal M, Cau P, Cremer H: Disruption of the mouse *Necdin* gene results in hypothalamic and behavioral alterations reminiscent of the human Prader-Willi syndrome. Hum Mol Genet 2000;9:3101–3110.
66 Mac Donald HR, Wevrick R: The necdin gene is deleted in Prader-Willi syndrome and is imprinted in human and mouse. Hum Mol Genet 1997;6:1873–1878.
67 Allen ND, Logan K, Lally G, Drage DJ, Norris ML, Keverne EB: Distribution of parthenogenetic cells in the mouse brain and their influence on brain development and behavior. Proc Natl Acad Sci USA 1995;92:10782–10786.
68 Keverne EB, Fundele R, Narasimha M, Barton SC, Surani MZ: Genomic imprinting and the differential roles of parental genomes in brain development. Dev Brain Res 1996;92:91–100.
69 Tilghman SM: The sins of the fathers and mothers: Genomic imprinting in mammalian development. Cell 1999;96:185–193.

Sergio R. Ojeda, DVM
Division of Neuroscience, Oregon National Primate Research Center/
Oregon Health & Science University
505 N.W. 185th Avenue, Beaverton, OR, 97006 (USA)
Tel. +1 503 690 5303, Fax +1 503 690 5384, E-Mail ojedas@ohsu.edu

Delemarre-van de Waal HA (ed): Abnormalities in Puberty. Scientific and Clinical Advances.
Endocr Dev. Basel, Karger, 2005, vol 8, pp 94–125

Gonadotropin-Releasing Hormone Analogue Treatment for Precocious Puberty

Twenty Years of Experience

Sabine Heger[a], *Wolfgang G. Sippell*[a], *Carl-Joachim Partsch*[b]

[a]Division of Paediatric Endocrinology, Department of Paediatrics, Christian-Albrechts-Universität, Universitätsklinikum Schleswig-Holstein, Campus Kiel, Kiel, and [b]Klinik für Kinder und Jugendliche, Städtische Kliniken, Esslingen, Germany

Abstract

Central precocious puberty (CPP) is the premature onset of puberty due to a precocious activation of gonadotropin-releasing hormone (GnRH) neurons in the hypothalamus. This condition results in accelerated development of secondary sex characteristics, accelerated bone maturation, impaired final height with disproportioned body appearance and can have a disturbing impact on the psychosocial behavior of children suffering from CPP. It is therefore necessary to assess the hormonal status of children who show pubertal signs before the age 8 years in girls and 9 years in boys. The indication for treatment should be made after evaluating pubertal progression, progression of bone age maturation and final height prognosis, development of reproductive function, and psychosocial adjustment and well-being. This paper summarizes the experience of GnRH agonist treatment, which is momentarily the treatment of choice for central precocious puberty in children.

Puberty is the transitional period in life during which the individual reaches sexual maturity and reproductive function. The initiation of puberty is due to events taking place in the central nervous system independently from the presence or absence of the gonads [1]. The result of these so far unknown events is the pulsatile secretion of gonadotropin-releasing hormone (GnRH) from a subset of highly specialized neurons located in the hypothalamus, which set in motion a cascade of downward events which finally lead to the production of gonadal sex steroids inducing the development of secondary sex characteristics and maintaining regular reproductive function in humans.

The premature activation of this cascade and the subsequent clinical appearance of precocious puberty have a profound impact on growth, development and psychosocial well-being of the patient. The outcome of untreated patients with precocious puberty is short stature, obesity and body disproportion [2–4]. In addition to psychosocial distress, the risks of sexual abuse [2, 5] and pregnancies in young children [6, 7] have been described.

After the introduction of short-acting GnRH agonists for the suppressive therapy of central precocious puberty (CPP) in 1981 [8], depot preparations of GnRH agonists have been available since the mid-1980s and have become the treatment of choice for CPP [9, 10]. Their suppressive effect on the pituitary-gonadal axis has been well documented, and its reversibility has been demonstrated [11, 12].

In this paper, we review some of the salient clinical, laboratory and radiological features of the possible causes of CPP and discuss current treatment options, monitoring requirements and long-term outcome.

Normal Puberty

Based on the large clinical trials performed by Marshall and Tanner [13, 14] in the United Kingdom at the end of the 1970s and Largo and Prader [15, 16] in Switzerland at the beginning of the 1980s, it has been generally accepted that approximately 95% of healthy girls start puberty with the enlargement of breasts (thelarche or stage B2) between 8.5 and 13 years of age. This stage is generally followed by pubic and axillary hair development. The mean start of puberty occurs around 11 years of age, the −2 SD limit is close to 9 years and the −3 SD limit close to 8 years of age. The age at which the appearance of secondary sex characteristics is considered to be normal in girls has been objected to discussion by a 1997 cross-sectional study of over 17,000 girls performed in the United States in a pediatric office setting [17]. According to this study based on mothers' reports and photographs, breast development occurred about 1 year earlier in Caucasian girls and 2 years earlier in African-American girls with a similar tendency for pubic hair development. Surprisingly, the age at menarche was not significantly different in Caucasian girls but 3 months advanced in African-American girls. However, a large cross-sectional survey performed in the Netherlands, investigating pubertal development from 1965 to 1997 did not observe this dramatic advancement of the onset of puberty [18]. Their observations, based on careful physical examination, demonstrated that 50% of girls had reached breast stage B2 at the age of 10.7 years and experienced menarche at 13.15 years of age. In boys the 50th percentile of pubertal stage G2 was reached at age 11.5 years [18].

Central Precocious Puberty

Definition

In girls, precocious puberty is generally defined as the appearance of thelarche before the age of 8 years. Menarche before the 9th birthday may serve as an additional criterion. In boys, the appearance of secondary sex characteristics before the 9th birthday is considered premature [19]. These diagnostic age thresholds were derived from studies investigating normal pubertal development and have a statistical basis which is somewhat arbitrarily chosen, since they are not equivalent to the generally applied age limits for the normal range as mentioned above (e.g. mean $\pm$ 2 SD). In addition, these diagnostic age limits may be subject to change over time [20], since the secular trend of advancement seems to continue in the future [21, 22]. The arbitrary nature of these age limits becomes clear when one considers that the diagnostic age limit for premature thelarche corresponds to approximately -2.5 to -3.0 SD below the normal mean age (10.9 $\pm$ 1.2 years [15]; 11.2 $\pm$ 1.1 years [13], 10.7 years [18]) and not to the usual limit of -2.0 SD. Even more pronounced is the cut-off age for menarche, in the range of -4 SD (11.32 years = 3rd centile, [23]; 11.77 = 10th centile, [21]). In addition, it is important to note that two percent of healthy girls may manifest pubertal stage B2 before their 8th birthday [15]. In boys the diagnostic age limit of 9 years for Tanner stage G2 corresponds to approximately -2.5 SD [14, 16, 24].

Incidence

Precocious puberty is a rare disorder, which occurs in approximately 1:5,000 to 1:10,000 children [25, 26] with a striking female gender preference of 3–23 to 1 (girls to boys) [27, 28]. Notably in boys neurological causes were as common as idiopathic CPP, whereas in girls neurological lesions were 5 times less common than idiopathic CPP [19, 28]. Thus, the risk of organic CPP is much higher in boys than in girls.

Etiology

The etiology of precocious puberty is variable and it is of utmost importance to distinguish between CPP which results from premature activation of the hypothalamic-pituitary-gonadal axis (GnRH-dependent) and GnRH-independent pseudoprecocious puberty [29, 30]. This distinction needs to be made in regard

Table 1. Etiology of central precocious puberty (gonadotropin dependent)

Category	Underlying disease
I. Permanent precocious puberty	
1. With abnormalities of the central nervous system	– hypothalamic hamartoma – *tumors:* astrocytoma, craniopharyngioma, ependymoma, glioma, LH-secreting adenoma, pinealoma – *congenital malformations:* arachnoid cyst, suprasellar cyst, phakomatosis, hydrocephalus (± spina bifida), septo-optic dysplasia – *acquired disease:* CNS infections, CNS abscess, radiation, chemotherapy, trauma
2. Without abnormalities of the central nervous system	
Precocious CNS maturation	– congenital adrenal hyperplasia – sex steroid-producing tumors – male-limited precocious puberty (familial or sporadic; constitutively activated LH receptor; e.g. Williams-Beuren syndrome) – adopted girls from developing countries
Idiopathic	– sporadic – familial
II. Transient precocious puberty	– idiopathic sporadic – arachnoid cyst – hydrocephalus

to diagnostic strategies and treatment strategies. Below we will focus on different etiologies of CPP and its variants (table 1).

Hypothalamic hamartomas are responsible for CPP in 2–28% of patients [29, 31]. These are congenital, non-neoplastic tumor-like lesions formed by heterotopic grey matter, neurons, glial cells and fiber bundles located at the base of the brain at the floor of the third ventricle, near to the tuber cinereum or to the mamillary bodies [32–35]. Hypothalamic hamartoma are more likely to cause precocious onset of pubertal development at a young age, usually <4 years [36–39] (fig. 1).

There is a predisposition for the development of CPP in children with neurofibromatosis type 1 [40, 41], in children with hydrocephalus [42, 43], meningomyelocele [44, 45], craniopharyngioma [46], neonatal encephalopathy [47], in children with chromosomal aberrations [48–50], and in children who have undergone low dose cranial irradiation [51, 52]. An association of Williams-Beuren syndrome with an increased frequency of CPP was recently

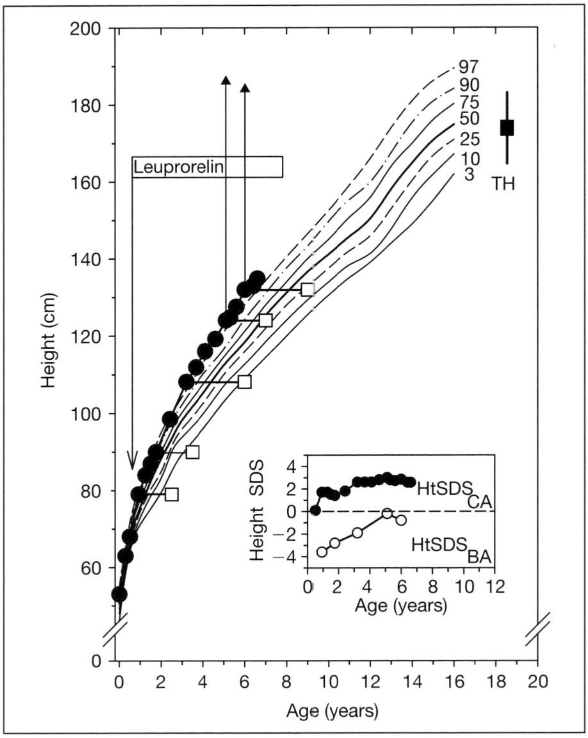

Fig. 1. Growth chart of a boy with central precocious puberty due to a hypothalamic hamartoma. Onset of puberty was at the very young age of 6 months. The patient had experienced a pubertal growth spurt between age 6 and 12 months when GnRH agonist treatment was started. CA = Chronological age (filled circle); BA = bone age (open square); PAH = predicted adult height (filled triangle); inset: SDS_{CA} = filled circle; SDS_{BA} = open circle.

reported [53–57]. Furthermore, early and precocious puberty is frequently observed in children adopted from developing countries. Improved nutritional, psychological and/or environmental conditions are thought to trigger the onset of puberty in these children [58–64].

In some cases, long-term exposure to sex steroids results in the maturation of central nervous system centers that are important for the initiation of puberty. The drop in sex steroids during treatment of the primary disease causes an activation of the prematurely matured hypothalamic GnRH pulse generator via feedback mechanisms, resulting in so-called secondary CPP. Thus, secondary CPP can occur after successful treatment of congenital adrenal hyperplasia [65–68], after removal of a sex steroid producing tumor [69–71] familial or sporadic male-limited precocious puberty [72–76] and has been described in a few patients with McCune-Albright syndrome [77, 78].

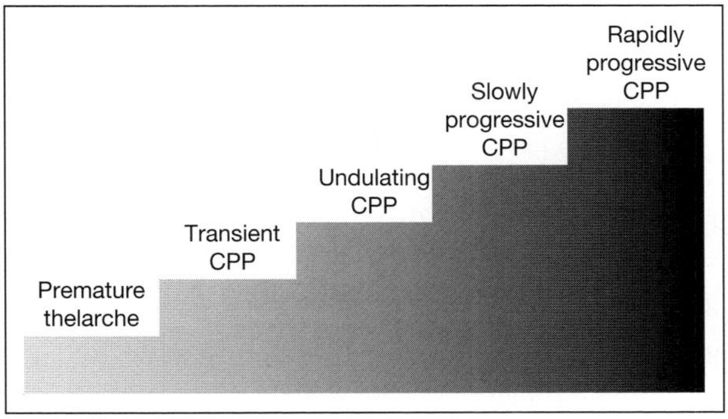

Fig. 2. Spectrum of precocious pubertal development.

As mentioned above, approximately 50% of the cases of CPP in boys and over 70% of the cases in girls remain so-called 'idiopathic' CPP. It is currently believed that increased GnRH secretion at the onset of puberty is a consequence of an increase in neuronal activity, also known as the central drive [79]. Two complementary mechanisms have been postulated to trigger this major event, one of them, known as the 'central restraint' of puberty, presumes that the tonic, inhibitory input affecting the GnRH network during childhood is lost at puberty. The second mechanism is the gain of excitatory inputs facilitating GnRH release at the time of puberty [19, 80]. A vast amount of research is underway to elucidate the neuroendocrine mechanisms controlling the normal initiation of puberty. GnRH neurons are affected by inhibitory and stimulatory inputs from different sources [81, 82]. It has become clear now that they are regulated by neurotransmitters, signalling peptides and growth factors communicating via neuron to neuron and glia to neuron communication networks [39, 80, 83–86]. It can be hypothesized that disturbances of the homeostasis of these functional networks could result in alterations to the time point of the onset of puberty, similar to those already demonstrated for delayed puberty [87, 88].

Course

Due to the sequence of hormonal events, CPP is usually consonant although there may be marked variations in the effect of sex steroids on the development of secondary sex characteristics, height velocity, bone maturation and psychosocial disturbances. Furthermore, partial or incomplete forms of precocious puberty (e.g. premature thelarche, premature pubarche) should be distinguished from complete forms, as should persistent from transient forms of CPP [30, 89] in order to avoid unnecessary treatment of these patients (fig. 2). In rapidly progressive CPP, pubertal development is highly accelerated and proceeds much faster than in normal puberty. Furthermore, the hormonal milieu is pathological: spontaneous LH pulses are of increased amplitude and plasma LH shows markedly increased levels after GnRH stimulation compared with the normal range for the respective pubertal stage [90, 91].

Diagnostic Evaluation

Clinical Signs/Auxology

The evaluation of a patient with CPP is based on the history of first manifestation of pubertal signs and how fast they progressed. A positive family history of precocious puberty may suggest familial cases of CPP, especially in cases of familial male precocious puberty. Growth rate over the last 6–12 months, presence of secondary sex characteristics and additional pubertal signs such as acne, oily skin, erections, nocturnal emissions in boys and vaginal discharge and menstrual bleedings in girls need to be assessed. Progression of pubertal maturation is usually increased in patients with CPP.

The physical examination includes the pubertal stages according to Tanner and the measurement of height, weight and body proportions. A growth curve including all available height data should be plotted (fig. 1). Height velocity is calculated on the basis of the available height data: most CPP patients have a height velocity >75th centile (fig. 3). An X-ray of the non-dominant (left) hand and wrist is taken to determine the biological age of the child. If the bone age (BA) is accelerated by more than 2 SD [177] for chronological age (CA), it is unlikely that the child has a normal variant of pubertal development. The SD of bone age is dependent on age and bone age [177]. The SD is between 7 and 11 months, and between 7 and 10 months for girls and boys aged 4–8 years, respectively [177]. In clinical practice, a bone advancement of more than 1 year can be taken as a significant acceleration in 4- to 8-year-old children. Whenever possible, the ratio of $\Delta BA/\Delta CA$ should be calculated during a pretreatment observation period. This ratio is over 1.2 in the majority of patients with progressive CPP [92].

Hormonal Findings

Plasma gonadotropin levels, gonadal steroid levels, frequency of luteinizing hormone (LH) pulses [93] and LH response to GnRH administration are within the pubertal range. The GnRH test is an important tool to distinguish between central true precocious puberty and pseudo-precocious GnRH-independent precocious puberty [90]. It has been demonstrated that it is sufficient to take only one blood sample after 30 min of GnRH administration [94]. Remarkably, the GnRH-stimulated LH concentration is not only higher than the prepubertal range but is also in excess of the normal range for the respective pubertal stage in 55% of girls with CPP [90].

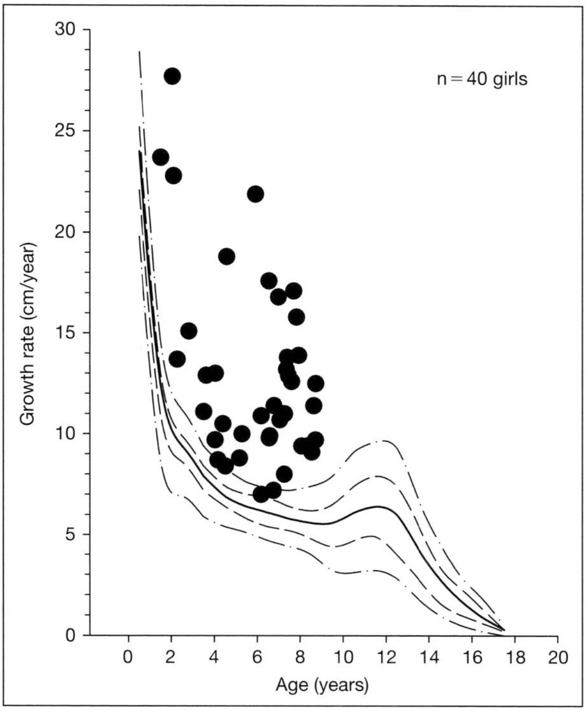

Fig. 3. Growth rate of 40 girls with central precocious puberty before treatment with depot GnRH agonist.

The rapid growth is associated with increased growth hormone secretion, and elevated IGF-1 and IGFBP3 levels can be detected in most children [95].

Additional laboratory investigations include thyroid function tests, 17-hydroxyprogesterone and hCG determination to exclude other causes of precocious puberty.

Imaging Techniques

All children with CPP should undergo magnetic resonance imaging (MRI) to rule out central nervous system (CNS) tumors or other CNS lesions as a cause of or associated with CPP [35, 96]. Recent studies have shown that CPP may be the only presenting symptom of an intracranial tumor or lesion [36, 96–98]. Restricting neuroradiological imaging to a certain subgroup of CPP patients, i.e. only boys or young girls, is not justified, because the occurrence of intracranial lesions has been demonstrated to be present in both sexes and all age groups [28, 36, 99].

Pelvic and abdominal ultrasound investigations are useful for two reasons, first to assess the enlargement of the uterus and ovaries caused by CPP and second to exclude other causes of sexual precocity, such as autonomous ovarian cysts or ovarian or adrenal neoplasms. The volumes of ovaries are important diagnostic sonographic parameters for CPP [100–102], in the case of CPP usually showing a bilateral enlargement of ovarian volume and development of macrocystic follicular structures [103, 104]. The volume of the uterus is increased and pear-shaped in contrast to a tubular shape in prepubertal children and in advanced cases the endometrium is clearly visible [102, 105–107].

Treatment of Central Precocious Puberty

Indications

There is no general consensus in the literature on the indication for treatment of CPP children [108–112]. However, there is consensus that not all patients with CPP may need medical suppression of the activity of the pituitary-gonadal axis [89, 109, 112]. The indication for treatment may be either for psychosocial and behavioral reasons or it may be for auxological reasons. A combination of both indication fields is also possible.

Psychosocial and Behavioral Aspects

Some psychological problems and long-term psychological sequelae have been described in CPP patients [6, 113] and early maturing girls [112, 114]. Two major concerns of parents with a child with CPP are the risks of sexual abuse and of early pregnancy [2, 5]. In fact, girls with early menarche consider themselves more mentally mature and they often peer up with older friends. Their relationship with parents and teachers is more critical and their school performance drops compared to their age peers [112, 114]. In patients with mental retardation and/or specific character traits, e.g. children with Williams-Beuren syndrome, early sexual activity, excessive masturbation and sexual aggression cause particular concern in both the families and the peer groups (e.g. kindergarten). While the psychosocial and behavioral aspects are completely ignored by several authors as potential indications for treatment in CPP [108, 109], we and others believe that these psychosocial/behavioral indications for treatment of CPP have to be considered individually together with the parents [111, 115]. Some general and evidence-based criteria are now available [113, 114] but will probably not be applicable in the individual case.

Auxological (Somatic) and Hormonal Aspects

There is much uncertainty regarding adequate criteria in regard to the auxological indication for treating children with CPP [110]. A specific bone age [110], or rapid advancement of bone age [109], or compromised predicted adult height [111] are stated by different authors as indications for treatment. To come to a minimum consensus, it is generally agreed that it is necessary to treat children with complete and progressive CPP in combination with some evidence for pubertal gonadotropin secretion and a pathological GnRH test. This implies that many children must undergo careful follow-up examinations before a decision on the indication for treatment can be made [109, 110]. In contrast to others [108, 111], our experience is that sex steroid levels are helpful in the decision-making process for or against treatment only if they are constantly elevated to the pubertal range [12, 16, 110]. Clear cut-off values do not exist [112].

We therefore suggest the following indications for treatment:

1. Complete precocious puberty and
2. Pubertal LH level after GnRH stimulation + peak LH/FSH ratio above diagnostic limit (e.g. 1.0) and
3. Rapid pubertal development (progression from one pubertal stage to the next in a markedly shorter period of time than normal) and
4. Abnormal height potential:
   - height prediction below the 3rd centile or
   - height prediction below target height range or
   - height SDS for bone age below −2.0 or
   - loss of height potential during follow-up and/or
5. Psychosocial reasons with:
   - behavioral disturbances or
   - emotional immaturity or
   - mental retardation or
   - specific personality patterns (e.g. as in Williams-Beuren syndrome)
   - menstrual hygiene in handicapped girls (e.g. meningo-myelocele).

GnRH agonist treatment is not indicated on auxological grounds in patients with no evidence of pubertal gonadotropin secretion and with slowly progressing CPP [30, 89, 109]. In the case of uncompromised or normal height potential additional indications should be present, otherwise treatment is not necessary [108, 110, 111].

Treatment Aims

Treatment goals are the maintenance of psychosocial well-being, prevention of early menarche and early sexual activity, regression of secondary sexual characteristics, avoidance of unfavorable body proportions, preservation of normal height potential within the target height range and diminishing the increased risk of breast cancer associated with early menarche [116].

Treatment Options

Three principle agents have been used in CPP therapy: medroxyprogersterone acetate (MPA), cyproterone acetate (CPA) and GnRH agonists. MPA and CPA reverse or arrest the progression of secondary sex characterises but have little to no effect on hormonal suppression [117, 118] and auxological outcome [4, 119]. In addition, both agents have undesirable side effects [4, 120].

With the availability of GnRH agonists, synthetic analogues of the natural GnRH decapeptide, MPA and CPA have become obsolete in the treatment of children with CPP. GnRH agonists bind to the GnRH receptor in the pituitary gland resulting in desensitization of the gonadotropins to GnRH and down-regulation of pituitary GnRH receptors [121, 122], so that gonadotropin release is gradually inhibited after an initial stimulatory phase ('flare-up') [123]. Additionally, GnRH agonist treatment leads to a disturbed transcription of LH α and β subunit gene. The β subunit amount decreases dramatically, the α subunit secretion is stimulated by exogenous GnRH administration [124], resulting in an ineffective LH.

The first reports of successful short-term pituitary-gonadal suppression in CPP patients by GnRH agonists date back to 1981 [8, 125, 126]. Since then numerous studies have been performed to investigate the psychological, hormonal and auxological effects of GnRH agonists in CPP children and to define the outcome after treatment.

Several GnRH agonists have been used in studies on treatment of CPP, since different compounds are licensed for the use in children in different countries. Routes and frequency of administration include 1–3 daily subcutaneous injections, multiple daily intranasal applications, and monthly intramuscular or subcutaneous depot injections.

Depot preparations of GnRH agonists [9] suppress the pituitary-hormonal axis far better than the daily subcutaneous or nasal preparations [127–129], probably due to improved patient compliance.

The most widely used drugs are triptorelin depot [9, 10, 130, 131] and leuprorelin depot [132–135]. Both leuprorelin depot and triptorelin depot were initially applied intramuscularly; however, these injections were very painful for the patients. Pharmacotechnological development has now made the considerably less painful subcutaneous route of administration possible for both compounds [135, 136].

The recommended dosage of triptorelin is 75–100 μg/kg body weight/4 weeks [9, 137], for leuprorelin a dose of 90 μg/kg body weight was shown to be efficacious for achieving pituitary-gonadal suppression [134, 138]. For practical reasons a starting dose of 3.75 mg (1 ampoule) for body weight ≥20 kg and 1.875 mg (1/2 ampoule) for body weight <20 kg is recommended in Europe [132, 136]. However, in the US a starting dose of 7.5 mg is used [133, 134]. Since no difference in long-term results between the European and the US patients has been demonstrated to date, we believe that the European dose should be used. Thus, a minimal injection volume (1 ml) can be administered, local reactions (e.g. sterile abscesses) can be reduced and treatment costs can be lowered.

Recently a 3-month depot formulation of leuprorelin has been developed [139] and licensed for prostate cancer [140]. In a couple of pilot studies the efficacy of this preparation for treating CPP has been successfully tested [141, 142] and has now been licensed for CPP in France and Italy. From the children's point of view it would be desirable to make treatment more convenient by lengthening the injection intervals.

Additionally, GnRH-receptor antagonists, which immediately block the effect of GnRH, have recently been developed for clinical use [143]. Currently, they serve as treatment in assisted reproduction. So far no clinical data exist to show whether these agents would also work in CPP, although animal experiments are encouraging [144, 145].

Treatment effects

3,155 publications are available under the key words precocious puberty in the electronic data base on scientific literature, Medline; however, only 26 can be found with the search limitation 'randomized controlled trial'. These numbers highlight the paucity of evidence-based studies in the field. Two of these 26 randomized studies deal with advanced or early-normal puberty [130, 146]. One study is about partial precocious puberty [129]. One study reports about the treatment of short children with GnRH agonists [147]. Three studies report on combined treatment with GnRH agonist and GH in patients with either CPP or early puberty [148–150], and two of these are on adopted children with early or precocious puberty [148, 150]. Two studies compare the effects of two different agonists in a randomized trial [128, 129], and one study deals with bone mass at final height, comparing the outcome with and without calcium supplementation [151]. It has to be accepted that no evidence-based data are available on the effects of treatment on hormonal suppression (exception [128]), on side effects and on outcome parameters such as final height (exception [128]), body proportions, bone mineral density (exception [151]), obesity, and psychosocial adjustment, psychosocial benefit or behavioral changes. A similar response to GnRH treatment has also been reported in adopted children with early onset of puberty [152].

Clinical, Hormonal and Psychological Effects

The suppressive effect of GnRH agonists on the pituitary-gonadal axis has been well documented in several studies [9, 91, 131]. As a consequence of the

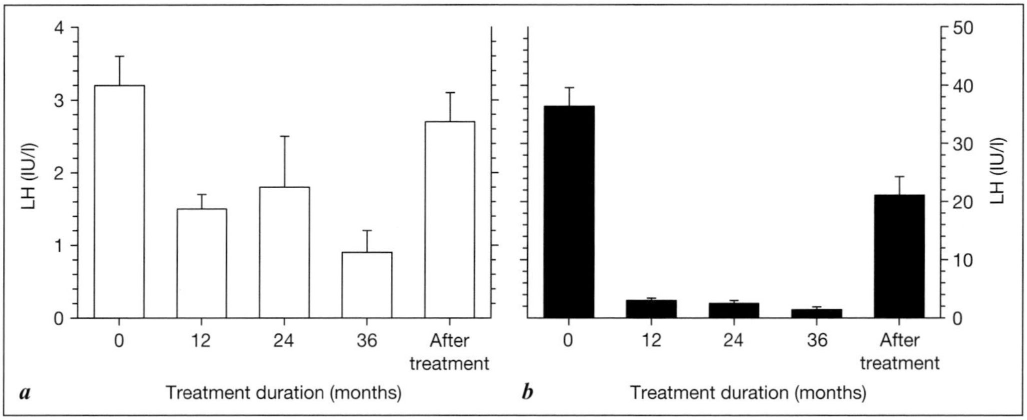

Fig. 4. Basal plasma LH levels (***a***), and after GnRH stimulation (***b***) in girls with central precocious puberty at diagnosis, during three years of treatment with the depot GnRH agonist triptorelin, and after recovery of the hypothalamic-pituitary-gonadal axis.

suppression of LH (fig. 4), estradiol and testosterone return to prepubertal levels [25, 94]. Reduction of breast size, pubic hair and ovarian and uterine size in girls, and decrease of testicular volumes in boys has been observed. Penile erections are less frequent and aggressive behavior, which occurs particularly in boys, shows a profound decrease in frequency and severity. Both boys and girls often show a remarkable improvement in terms of attention and school performance.

Auxological Effects

Height velocity and bone maturation rate are reduced in both sexes. The gap between height SDS for CA and height SDS for BA decreases continuously during treatment (fig. 5). The auxological effect of long-term depot GnRH agonist treatment is shown in figures 1, 5 and 6.

Side Effects

Due to the mode of action of GnRH agonists, LH and sex steroids increase in the initial phase of treatment ('flare-up phase') following the first injection of the agonist. The stimulation of LH and estradiol or testosterone lasts for at least 4 days [153]. Following this, transient vaginal withdrawal bleedings may occur in girls [9, 135, 154].

In one study, prolonged and recurrent vaginal bleeding in 8 of 28 patients treated with triptorelin depot was observed [155], however we did not see this side effect in two large multicenter trials [91, 131]. Further side effects include

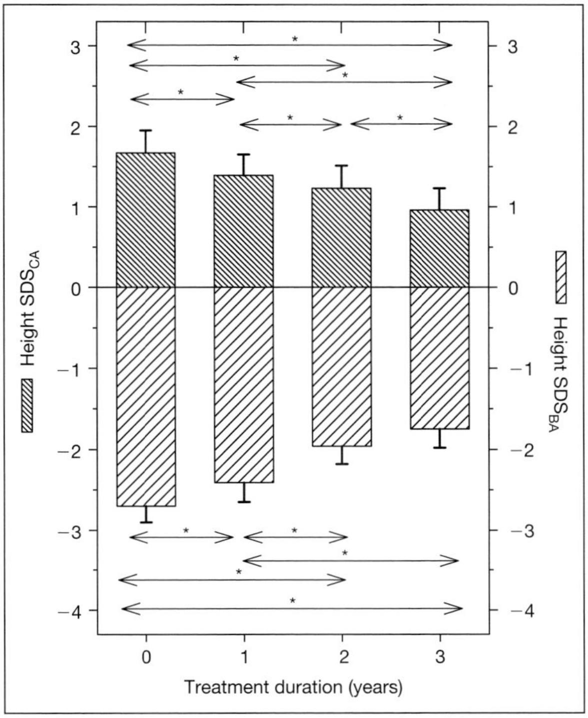

Fig. 5. Longitudinal growth data of 24 girls with progressive central precocious puberty. Height standard deviation score (SDS) for chronological age (CA; upper panel, mean ± SEM) and height SDS for bone age (BA, lower panel, mean ± SEM) before treatment with a depot GnRH agonist (leuprorelin acetate) and during the first 3 years of treatment. * $p < 0.05$.

minor menopausal symptoms in girls (e.g. head ache, nausea, hot flushes in 2–5% of patients) and local allergic reactions in up to 10% of patients [135, 141, 142], as well as the formation of sterile abscesses at the injection site in both sexes [132, 133, 156–158]. In our experience the risk of a sterile abscess increases with the injection dose and volume and is greater when injected in the abdomen than in the thigh. While a prospective, double-blind placebo-controlled study showed an increase in depressive mood symptoms in women treated with GnRH agonists for endometriosis [159], no such study is available in girls (or boys) with CPP. Weight gain during GnRH agonist treatment has been of particular concern to the patients and their families. Obesity after end of treatment has been reported in patients with hypothalamic hamartoma [160]; however, an increased BMI SDS was already present in these patients at diagnosis [91]. It has been demonstrated that GnRH agonists do not cause obesity during treatment [91, 161, 162]. The development of body mass index during

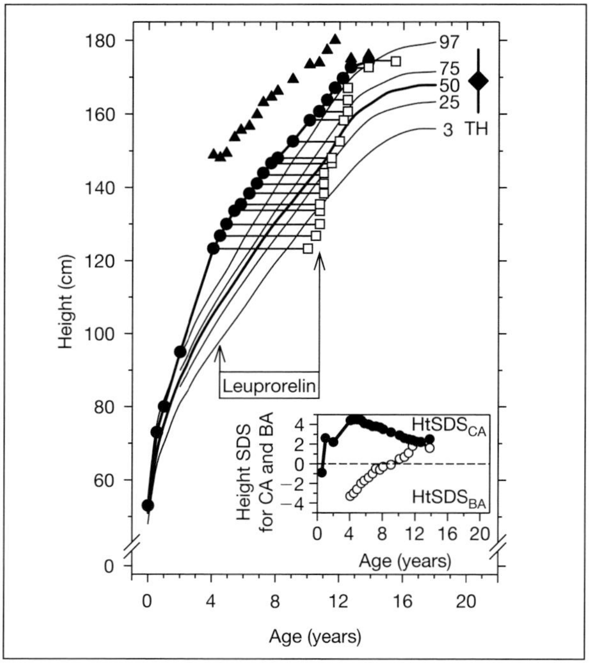

Fig. 6. Growth chart of a girl with idiopathic central precocious puberty and onset of puberty at age 2 years. CA = Filled circle; BA = open square; PAH = filled triangle; inset: SDS_{CA} = filled circle, SDS_{BA} = open circle.

GnRH agonist treatment is shown in figure 7. Antibody formation against the agonist has not been reported, even in patients with allergic skin reactions [163]. In general, the side effects of GnRH agonist treatment in children are of minor severity and acceptable [91, 164].

Monitoring Treatment

In most patients a halt or involution of secondary sex characteristics, uterus and ovarian size, growth rate, and bone maturation can be observed after initiation of therapy.

To monitor these effects clinical examination with determination of pubertal stages and measurement of height, weight and body proportions at regular 3-monthly intervals during the first treatment year and at 6 monthly intervals thereafter are indicated. Height velocity must be calculated at yearly intervals to ensure normal growth and to indicate pathological growth deceleration with

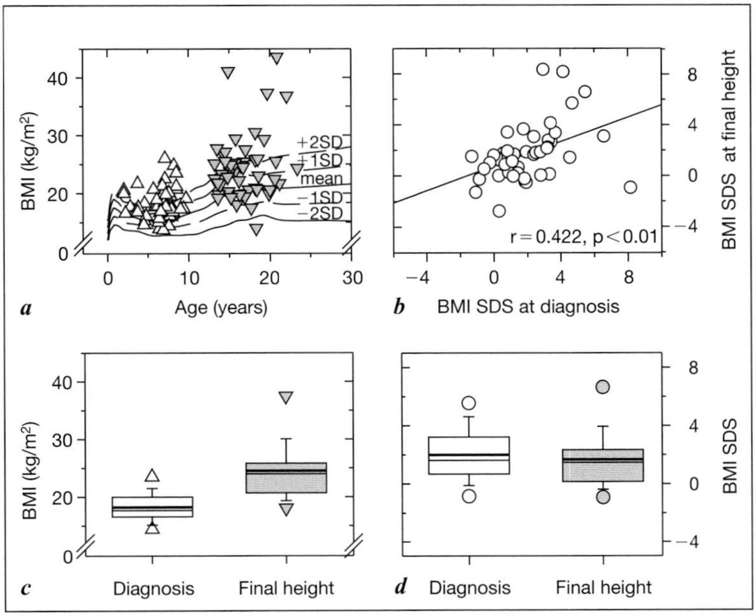

Fig. 7. Panel ***a*** and ***c*** body mass index (BMI) at diagnosis of precocious puberty (white triangles) and at final height (grey triangles). ***b*** Relationship of BMI expressed as standard deviation score (SDS) at time of diagnosis and at final height, demonstrating that GnRH agonist treatment per se does not cause girls with precocious puberty to become obese. Panel ***d*** BMI SDS at diagnosis of precocious puberty (white circles) and at final height (grey circles); light line, median; heavy line, mean; circles, 5th to 95th percentile.

the possible need for additional growth-promoting treatment. In addition, bone age evaluation is necessary in at least yearly intervals in order to estimate any changes in height potential (height SDS for bone age, PAH; fig. 6)

The most useful single test to ensure adequate suppression of the hypothalamic-pituitary-gonadal axis is the GnRH stimulation of LH release [165]. If the recommended injection interval and the recommended dosage for depot GnRH agonist preparations are strictly adhered to, a sufficient suppression of GnRH-stimulated LH can be expected in all patients after varying durations of therapy (fig. 4) [91, 131, 132, 154]. However, in some patients an increase in GnRH agonist dosage may be necessary in order to achieve suppression [132, 135].

Several alternatives to the i.v. GnRH stimulation test have been proposed. In the single sample subcutaneous GnRH stimulation test one blood sample is drawn for LH determination 40 min after s.c. injection of 100 μg GnRH [166]. There was a fairly good correlation between peak LH after i.v. and s.c. GnRH ($r = 0.88$, $p < 0.0001$). Validation of this test yielded favorable results. As a second alternative to the standard i.v. GnRH test, a single blood sample taken 12 h after the injection of the GnRH agonist for determination of LH, FSH and estradiol may be used to monitor pituitary-gonadal suppression [153]. The advantages of this test are (a) a single blood sample is sufficient, no iv line is necessary; (b) GnRH can be saved, thus costs are reduced; (c) not only the pituitary response but also the ovarian response (plasma estradiol increase) is tested (additional information that may help to identify non responders or poor responders early). However, the 12-hour interval may not be compatible with outpatient settings in all places. The monitoring of girls during treatment solely by following plasma estradiol levels is considered inadequate because of overlapping plasma levels between prepubertal and pubertal girls; girls with CPP have prepubertal estradiol levels in up to 50% of cases before treatment [135], and because of marked intra-individual variations. In boys a low morning plasma testosterone level below 35 ng/dl is a clear indication of adequate suppression [165]. A puberty suppression score which includes clinical, hormonal, and auxological parameters has been proposed to evaluate GnRH agonist-induced suppression [167], but this score has several inherent problems and has not found its way into clinical routine. To date, the use of urinary gonadotropin determination has been proven itself to be an adequate replacement for the GnRH stimulation test [168, 169].

The involution of enlarged ovarian volumes [102–104] and uterus volume and shape [102, 105] are monitored by ultrasound. Ovarian volume and uterine volume return to the normal range within 3 to 12 months of treatment [9, 132, 170]. However, these parameters should neither be used as the only diagnostic tool for identifying CPP patients nor as the only tool for monitoring treatment [171].

Final Outcome

Pituitary and Gonadal Function

Complete reversibility of suppression of the hypothalamic-pituitary-gonadal axis after discontinuation of GnRH agonist therapy has been demonstrated [12, 91, 95, 104, 172]. It is important to note that there is a further maturation of the GnRH pulse generator during GnRH agonist treatment [173]. Thus, the levels of gonadotropins, the pulsatile characteristics of gonadotropin secretion, and the levels of sex steroids reach a late pubertal state within a short period of time after the end of GnRH agonist treatment [173, 174]. This explains why menarche occurs within a few months after stopping treatment in many girls [11, 12, 91, 173, 174]. In terms of gonadal function and morphology, discrepant results are reported in the literature. One study reported an increased prevalence of polycystic ovaries in CPP girls who received combined treatment with GnRH agonist and GH [103]; however, PCO-like ovaries were seen only rarely or not at all in studies with GnRH agonists alone [91, 104, 170]. Furthermore, the clinical significance of polycystic ovaries on ultrasound in young women without reproductive problems is still unclear [174]. Although data on large numbers of former patients are not yet available, our own experience (normal pregnancies with 5 healthy children in over 50 former CPP patients) and that of other centers indicate that fertility and pregnancy outcome are probably normal, even after prolonged GnRH agonist treatment (up to 10 years in our series). Correspondingly, there is an indication that spermatogenesis is unaffected after GnRH agonist treatment in boys, once the pituitary-gonadal axis has recovered from hormonal suppression. These human data are in accordance with results from several animal studies which show that spermatogenesis recovers completely after long-term GnRH agonist treatment in juvenile and adult primates [144].

Final Height

To date, a considerable number of CPP patients who were treated with various GnRH agonists over many years have reached final height (FH) and adult age. The long-term outcome with respect to final height is summarized in table 2 for girls and in table 3 for boys. It has now become clear that treatment with GnRH agonists, particularly when administered as depot preparation, preserves adult height potential, and that adult height is increased in most studies of girls with CPP compared to untreated patients as well as to individual height prediction before treatment (for example, see fig. 6). While there are no randomized studies available in the literature which report final height in CPP patients, four studies reported on final height in advanced or early normal puberty [130, 146, 175, 176]. From these reports it is clear that GnRH agonists do not improve mean final height in girls over 8 years of age at start of treatment (with a mean bone age of 10.9, 10.6, 9.97 and 12.6 years, respectively).

When final heights are compared to initial height predictions, the results are less positive in boys with CPP than in girls (table 3). However, results are impressively positive when compared with untreated patients. This discrepancy is most probably due to the methodological problems and limitations of adult height prediction in children with CPP. In fact, the height prediction methods most widely used in clinical practice [177–179] have not been validated in large numbers of patients with CPP. However, in the absence of a prediction alternative the Bayley-Pinneau method has been investigated for its application to patients with CPP [180–182]. These studies clearly showed that final height is overestimated in CPP patients by up to 13 cm. The use of the B&P tables for average girls and boys instead of those for children with accelerated bone age resulted in more accurate height predictions [181, 182] (tables 2, 3).

Therefore, the inaccuracy of adult height predictions and the remaining over-prediction with the use of the average tables should be taken into account

Table 2. Survey of final height of girls with central precocious puberty or early normal puberty without treatment or with treatment by progestational agents or by various GnRH agonists

Reference	n	PAH cm	Final height cm	Target height cm	Treatment
Untreated					
Thamdrup, 1961 [2]	15	–	150.5	–	none
Sigurjonsdottir and Hayles, 1968 [3]	21	–	153.2	–	none
Werder et al., 1974 [119]	7	–	154.0	161.8	none
Lee, 1981 [193]	15	156.3	155.3	164.3	none
Schoevaart et al., 1990 [192]	8	–	161.7	–	none
Brauner et al., 1994 [194]	15	162.5	162.0	161.1	none (SP)
Stasiowska et al., 1994 [195]	10	–	149.8	153.3	none (control)
Antoniazzi et al., 1994 [128]	10	153.3	149.6	156.4	none (control)
Paul et al., 1995 [196]	8	–	153.8	–	none
Kauli et al., 1997 [181]	28	161.4	155.5	159.3	none (control)
Bertelloni et al., 1998 [188]	9	163.1	161.8	161.0	none (SP)
Bouvattier et al., 1999 [130]	10	155.2	156.1	157.8	none (SP)
Cassio et al., 1999 [146]	23	159.3	158.6	158.5	none (EP)
Palmert et al., 1999 [89]	20	–	165.5	164.0	none (SP)
Lazar et al., 2002 [175]	63	152.7	156.6	157.9	none (EP)
Progestational agents					
– CPA or MPA					
Lee, 1981 [193]	13	153.2	155.6	164.0	MPA
Sorgo et al., 1987 [4]	11	157.1	153.1	161.0	CPA
Schoevaart et al., 1990 [192]	16	–	162.2	–	CPA
Kato et al., 1993 [197]	16	–	151.3	155.4	CPA
Kauli et al., 1997 [181]	27	156.8	157.6	155.8	CPA
GnRH agonists					
– Daily s.c. or i.n.					
Boepple et al., 1991 [198]	27	147.5	149.9	–	Des/His s.c.
Oerter et al., 1991 [183]	38	151.8	157.0	165*	Des s.c.
Antoniazzi et al., 1994 [128]	15	152.9	153.2	155.5	Bus i.n.
Cacciari et al., 1994 [199]	12	156.7	159.5	162.5	Bus i.n.
Stasiowska et al., 1994 [195]	12	–	157.3	155.6	Bus s.c.
Klein et al., 2001 [200]	80	149.3	159.8	163.7	Des/His s.c.
GnRH agonists					
– Depot (i.m. or s.c.)					
Kauli et al., 1990 [201]	8	145.3	151.2	–	Tripto
Brauner et al., 1994 [194]	19	152.1	159.0	160.2	Tripto
Antoniazzi et al., 1994 [128]	15	154.1	160.6	157.6	Tripto
Paul et al., 1995 [196]	26	–	160.5	–	Naf/Des/Leupro
Oostdijk et al., 1996 [137]	31	158.2	161.6	168.7	Tripto

Table 2 (continued)

Reference	n	PAH cm	Final height cm	Target height cm	Treatment
Kauli et al., 1997 [181]	48	156.6	159.6	157.7	Tripto
Bertelloni et al., 1998 [188]	14	153.5	158.1	161.0	Bus→Tripto
Galluzzi et al., 1998 [202]	22	155.2	158.5	163.5	Tripto
Arrigo et al., 1999 [185]	71	155.5	158.4	161.5	Tripto
Carel et al., 1999 [203]	58	156.4	161.1	160.1	Tripto
Cassio et al., 1999 [146]	23	157.8	158.1	157.0	Tripto (EP)
Heger et al., 1999 [91]	50	154.9	160.6	163.6	Tripto
Mul et al., 2000 [204]	87	155.3§	162.5	168*	Tripto
Lazar et al., 2002 [175]	63	152.9	157.2	157.7	Tripto
Kempers et al., 2002 [152]	17	164.2	166.2	168.1	Tripto
Antoniazzi et al., 2003 [151]	48	152.9	159.9	161.9	Tripto
Pucarelli et al., 2003 [205]	18	153.9	156.6	157.2	Tripto
Lanes et al., 2004 [208]	8	153.6	162.6	157.4	Tripto/Leupro
Paterson et al., 2004 [209]	11	–	159.7	160.9	Goserelin

EP = Early puberty (7.5–8.5 years); SP = slowly progressive precocious puberty; CPA = cyproterone acetate; MPA = medroxyprogesterone acetate; Bus = buserelin; Des = deslorelin; His = histrelin; Leupro = leuprorelin; Naf = nafarelin; Tripto = triptorelin; control = control group from a treatment trial (see corresponding reference in another part of the table). * Taken from figure in reference no. 183 and 204, § average tables [177].

when interpreting height gain data in CPP patients. In addition, the last height prediction during treatment certainly over-estimates final height and patients will not grow to this calculated height [12, 91, 183] (fig. 6).

Even more important than the overall group data is the benefit of treatment to the individual. With depot GnRH agonist treatment, more than 75% of female CPP patients will reach their genetic target height range [91], approximately 40% will reach their individual target height, and more than 90% of patients will have a final height > 150 cm [181, 184–186]. These figures are clearly superior to untreated patients or those treated with CPA [181]. The main reasons for the lack of favorable final height results in some patients are the compromised height potential at start of treatment, i.e. patients are presented too late in the course of their precocious pubertal development or CPP patients borne short for gestational age (SGA) and additional familial factors (in many patients a component of familial short stature is found).

In contrast to the unfavorable body proportions with inappropriately short legs and arms seen in untreated patients [2], proportions are normal after GnRH agonist treatment at final height [91].

Table 3. Survey of final height of boys with progressive CPP after treatment with GnRH agonists or untreated

Reference	n	PAH cm	Final height cm	Target height cm	Treatment
Without treatment					
Thamdrup, 1961 [2]	8	–	155.4	–	none
Sigurjonsdottir and Hayles, 1968 [3]	14	–	156.1	–	none
Paul et al., 1995 [196]	23	–	155.6	–	none
GnRH agonists					
– Daily s.c. or i.n.					
Oerter et al., 1991 [183]	6	161.3	168.0	180*	Des
Paul et al., 1995 [196]	6	172.8	166.3	–	Naf/Des/Leu
Klein et al., 2001 [200]	18	156.1	171.1	178.3	Des/His
GnRH agonists					
– Depot i.m. or s.c.					
Oostdijk et al., 1996 [137]	5	177.4	171.5	178*	Tripto
Galluzzi et al., 1998 [202]	11	168.3	175.5	174.5	Tripto
Carel et al., 1999 [203]	8	174.2	172.8	171.8	Tripto
Mul et al., 2000 [204]	9	171.5§	170.8	179*	Tripto
Rizzo et al., 2000 [206]	12	169.9	176.1	174.2	Bus→Tripto
Lazar et al., 2001 [182]	11	174*§	172.3	170.6	Tripto
Mul et al., 2002 [207]	26	166*	172.9	176*	Tripto

Bus = Buserelin; Des = deslorelin; His = histrelin; Leu = leuprorelin; Naf = nafarelin; Tripto = triptorelin. * Taken from figure in references, § average tables [177].

Bone Mineral Density

Bone mineral density (BMD) is often increased for chronological age at diagnosis of CPP and then declines during agonist treatment [151, 187, 188] or remains unchanged [189]. However, in the long-term, BMD remains within the normal range in female patients at final height [91, 151, 188–190]. Thus, GnRH agonist treatment does not cause osteopenia or osteoporosis.

Body Weight

Many children with CPP are significantly overweight at first presentation: 48% with BMI SDS above 85th centile [161], 40% with BMI SDS above +2.0 [91, 162]. However, BMI SDS did not change significantly within the patient groups during treatment (fig. 7). At the last visit, off treatment, 44% of patients showed a BMI SDS >85th centile [161] and 31% still had a BMI SDS >2.0 (fig. 7). There was a significant correlation between BMI SDS at diagnosis and at final height. The strongest predictor of an elevated BMI SDS after treatment was the BMI SDS before treatment. Thus, it has now been clearly demonstrated that GnRH agonists do not cause obesity, but rather that children with CPP are prone to be overweight and obese from the start [91, 161].

Psychosocial Outcome

No evidence-based material is available with respect to psychosocial adjustment and outcome. Some studies suggest that precocious development can lead to specific behavioral problems in the patients such as negative feelings about their own physical appearance [191], and that patients with a risk factor may need psychosocial support [114]; others report no negative effect of early maturation on psychosocial well-being later in life [191]. All our female patients (n = 50) reported a good quality of life. None was unemployed or had dropped out of the educational system [91]. The psychological evaluation of adopted children with early puberty did not reveal any consistent abnormalities [113].

Conclusion

Since the management of CPP patients involves clinical, hormonal, sonographic and radiological aspects, expertise in all these areas is necessary to establish the diagnosis without delay and to make a judgment on the prognosis. The decision for or against treatment has to be made on an individual basis, and may require an observation period of 6–12 months to define the rate of progression of CPP. Depot GnRH agonists have now proven themselves to be the treatment of choice for this condition, resulting in effective suppression of pituitary-gonadal function in practically all patients. Side effects are of minor severity and are acceptable, rendering long-term treatment in young children with CPP both feasible and well tolerated. Hormonal suppression is fully reversed when treatment ends and there are no severe long-term sequelae of GnRH agonist treatment. In particular, fertility seems not to be compromised. It is possible that future developments will see the application of GnRH antagonists in the treatment of precocious puberty, in order to avoid the biological effect of the initial flare-up phase caused by GnRH agonists; however, antagonistic compounds are not yet available as depot preparations, which is a prerequisite for their use in children.

Acknowledgements

We are grateful to Joanna Voerste for linguistic help with the manuscript.

References

1 Wildt L, Marshall G, Knobil E: Experimental induction of puberty in the infantile rhesus monkey. Science 1980;207:1373–1375.
2 Thamdrup E: Precocious sexual development: A clinical study of one hundred children. Dan Med Bull 1961;8:140–142.
3 Sigurjonsdottir TJ, Hayles AB: Precocious puberty. A report of 96 cases. Am J Dis Child 1968;115:309–321.
4 Sorgo W, Kiraly E, Homoki J, Heinze E, Teller WM, Bierich JR, et al: The effects of cyproterone acetate on statural growth in children with precocious puberty. Acta Endocrinol (Copenh) 1987;115:44–56.
5 Herman-Giddens ME, Sandler AD, Friedman NE: Sexual precocity in girls. An association with sexual abuse? Am J Dis Child 1988;142:431–433.
6 Ehrhardt AA, Meyer-Bahlburg HF, Bell JJ, Cohen SF, Healey JM, Stiel R, et al: Idiopathic precocious puberty in girls: Psychiatric follow-up in adolescence. J Am Acad Child Psychiatry 1984;23:23–33.
7 Stoeckel H: Geburtshilfe, ed 5. Jena, VEB Thieme Verlag, 1938.
8 Crowley WF Jr, Comite F, Vale W, Rivier J, Loriaux DL, Cutler GB Jr: Therapeutic use of pituitary desensitization with a long-acting LhRH agonist: A potential new treatment for idiopathic precocious puberty. J Clin Endocrinol Metab 1981;52:370–372.
9 Roger M, Chaussain JL, Berlier P, Bost M, Canlorbe P, Colle M, et al: Long term treatment of male and female precocious puberty by periodic administration of a long-acting preparation of D-Trp6-luteinizing hormone-releasing hormone microcapsules. J Clin Endocrinol Metab 1986; 62:670–677.
10 Hümmelink R, Oostdijk W, Partsch CJ, Odink RJ, Drop SL, Sippell WG: Growth, bone maturation and height prediction after three years of therapy with the slow release GnRH-agonist decapeptyl-depot in children with central precocious puberty. Horm Metab Res 1992;24:121–126.
11 Manasco PK, Pescovitz OH, Feuillan PP, Hench KD, Barnes KM, Jones J, et al: Resumption of puberty after long term luteinizing hormone-releasing hormone agonist treatment of central precocious puberty. J Clin Endocrinol Metab 1988;67:368–372.
12 Oostdijk W, Partsch CJ, Drop SL, Sippell WG: Hormonal evaluation during and after long-term treatment with a slow-release GnRH-agonist of children with central precocious puberty; effect on final height; in Plant T, Lee PA (eds): The Neurobiology of Puberty. Bristol, Journal of Endocrinology, 1995, pp 319–325.
13 Marshall WA, Tanner JM: Variations in the pattern of pubertal changes in girls. Arch Dis Child 1969;44:291–303.
14 Marshall WA, Tanner JM: Variations in the pattern of pubertal changes in boys. Arch Dis Child 1970;45:13–23.
15 Largo RH, Prader A: Pubertal development in Swiss girls. Helv Paediatr Acta 1983;38:229–243.
16 Largo RH, Prader A: Pubertal development in Swiss boys. Helv Paediatr Acta 1983;38:211–228.
17 Herman-Giddens ME, Slora EJ, Wasserman RC, Bourdony CJ, Bhapkar MV, Koch GG, et al: Secondary sexual characteristics and menses in young girls seen in office practice: A study from the pediatric research in office settings network. Pediatrics 1997;99:505–512.
18 Mul D, Fredriks AM, van Buuren S, Oostdijk W, Verloove-Vanhorick SP, Wit JM: Pubertal development in The Netherlands 1965–1997. Pediatr Res 2001;50:479–486.
19 Grumbach MM, Styne DM: Puberty: Ontogeny, neuroendocrinology, physiology, and disorders; in Williams RH, Foster DW, Kroenenberg H, Larsen PR, Zorab R (eds): Williams Textbook of Endocrinology, ed 9. Philadelphia, Saunders, 1998, pp 1509–1625.
20 Kaplowitz PB, Oberfield SE: Reexamination of the age limit for defining when puberty is precocious in girls in the United States: Implications for evaluation and treatment. Pediatrics 1999;104: 936–941.
21 Fredriks AM, van Buuren S, Burgmeijer RJ, Meulmeester JF, Beuker RJ, Brugman E, et al: Continuing positive secular growth change in The Netherlands 1955–1997. Pediatr Res 2000; 47:316–323.

22 de Muinck Keizer-Schrama SMPF, Mul D: Trends in pubertal development in Europe. Hum Reprod Update 2001;7:287–291.
23 Engelhardt L, Willers B, Pelz L: Sexual maturation in East German girls. Acta Paediatr 2004;84: 1362–1365.
24 Willers B, Engelhardt L, Pelz L: Sexual maturation in East German boys. Acta Paediatr 1996;85:785–788.
25 Gonzalez ER: For puberty that comes too soon, new treatment highly effective. JAMA 1982;248: 1149–1152.
26 Cutler GB Jr: Precocious puberty; in Hurst JW (ed): Medicine for the Practicing Physician. Woburn, Butterworth, 1988, pp 526–530.
27 Kappy MS, Ganong CS: Advances in the treatment of precocious puberty. Adv Pediatr 1994;41: 223–261.
28 Bridges NA, Christopher JA, Hindmarsh PC, Brook CG: Sexual precocity: Sex incidence and aetiology. Arch Dis Child 1994;70:116–118.
29 Partsch CJ, Sippell WG: Pathogenesis and epidemiology of precocious puberty. Effects of exogenous oestrogens. Hum Reprod Update 2001;7:292–302.
30 Partsch CJ, Peter M, Heger S, Sippell WG: Self-remitting or transient central precocious puberty. Monatsschr Kinderheilkd 1998;146:678–682.
31 De Sanctis V, Corrias A, Rizzo V, Bertelloni S, Urso I, Galluzzi F, et al: Etiology of central precocious puberty in males: The results of the Italian Study Group for Physiopathology of Puberty. J Pediatr Endocrinol Metab 2000;13:693.
32 Starceski PJ, Lee PA, Albright AL, Migeon CJ: Hypothalamic hamartomas and sexual precocity. Am J Dis Child 1990;144:225–228.
33 Jung H, Carmel P, Schwartz MS, Witkin JW, Bentele KHP, Westphal M, et al: Some hypothalamic hamartomas contain transforming growth factor alpha, a puberty-inducing growth factor, but not luteinizing hormone-releasing hormone neurons. J Clin Endocrinol Metab 1999;84:4695–4701.
34 Jung H, Neumaier Probst E, Hauffa BP, Partsch CJ, Dammann O: Association of morphological characteristics with precocious puberty and/or gelastic seizures in hypothalamic hamartoma. J Clin Endocrinol Metab 2003;88:4590–4595.
35 Brandberg G, Raininko R, Eeg-Olofsson O: Hypothalamic hamartoma with gelastic seizures in Swedish children and adolescents. Eur J Paediatr Neurol 2004;8:35–44.
36 Cisternino M, Arrigo T, Pasquino AM, Tinelli C, Antoniazzi F, Beduschi L, et al: Etiology and age incidence of precocious puberty in girls: A multicentric study. J Pediatr Endocrinol Metab 2000;13:695–701.
37 Comite F, Pescovitz OH, Rieth KG, Dwyer AJ, Hench K, McNemar A, et al: Luteinizing hormone-releasing hormone analog treatment of boys with hypothalamic hamartoma and true precocious puberty. J Clin Endocrinol Metab 1984;59:888–892.
38 Mahachoklertwattana P, Kaplan SL, Grumbach MM: The luteinizing hormone-releasing hormone-secreting hypothalamic hamartoma is a congenital malformation: Natural history. J Clin Endocrinol Metab 1993;77:118–124.
39 Ojeda SR, Prevot V, Heger S, Dziedzic B: Gonadotropin-releasing hormone and puberty; in Henry HL, Norman AW (eds): Encyclopedia of Hormones. San Diego, Academic Press, 2003, pp 165–171.
40 Carmi D, Shohat M, Metzker A, Dickerman Z: Growth, puberty, and endocrine functions in patients with sporadic or familial neurofibromatosis type 1: A longitudinal study. Pediatrics 1999;103:1257–1262.
41 Virdis R, Sigorini M, Laiolo A, Lorenzetti E, Street ME, Villani AR, et al: Neurofibromatosis type 1 and precocious puberty. J Pediatr Endocrinol Metab 2000;13:844–847.
42 De Luca F, Muritano M, Rizzo G, Pandullo E, Cardia E: True precocious puberty: A long-term complication in children with shunted non-tumoral hydrocephalus. Helv Paediatr Acta 1985;40:467–472.
43 Lopponen T, Saukkonen AL, Serlo W, Tapanainen P, Ruokonen A, Knip M: Accelerated pubertal development in patients with shunted hydrocephalus. Arch Dis Child 1996;74:490–496.
44 Meyer S, Landau H: Precocious puberty in myelomeningocele patients. J Pediatr Orthop 1984; 4:28–31.
45 Trollmann R, Dörr HG, Strehl E, Katalinic A, Beyer R, Wenzel D: Growth and pubertal development in patients with meningomyelocele: A retrospective analysis. Acta Paediatr 1996;85:76–80.

46 de Vries L, Lazar L, Phillip M: Craniopharyngioma: Presentation and endocrine sequelae in 36 children. J Pediatr Endocrinol Metab 2003;16:703–710.
47 Robertson CM, Morrish DW, Wheler GH, Grace MG: Neonatal encephalopathy: An indicator of early sexual maturation in girls. Pediatr Neurol 1990;6:102–108.
48 Grosso S, Balestri P, Anichini C, Bartalini G, Pucci L, Morgese G, et al: Pubertal disorders in inv dup(15) syndrome. Gynecol Endocrinol 2001;15:165–169.
49 Grosso S, Berardi R, Pucci L, Balestri P: Precocious puberty with trisomy X syndrome. Obstet Gynecol 1999;94:861.
50 Fokstuen S, Ginsburg C, Zachmann M, Schinzel A: Maternal uniparental disomy 14 as a cause of intrauterine growth retardation and early onset of puberty. J Pediatr 1999;134:689–695.
51 Brauner R, Czernichow P, Rappaport R: Precocious puberty after hypothalamic and pituitary irradiation in young children. N Engl J Med 1984;311:920.
52 Ogilvy-Stuart AL, Clayton PE, Shalet SM: Cranial irradiation and early puberty. J Clin Endocrinol Metab 1994;78:1282–1286.
53 Cherniske EM, Sadler LS, Schwartz D, Carpenter TO, Pober BR: Early puberty in Williams syndrome. Clin Dysmorphol 1999;8:117–121.
54 Partsch CJ, Dreyer G, Gosch A, Winter M, Schneppenheim R, Wessel A, et al: Longitudinal evaluation of growth, puberty, and bone maturation in children with Williams syndrome. J Pediatr 1999;134:82–89.
55 Scothorn DJ, Butler MG: How common is precocious puberty in patients with Williams syndrome? Clin Dysmorphol 1997;6:91–93.
56 Partsch CJ, Japing I, Siebert R, Gosch A, Wessel A, Sippell WG, et al: Central precocious puberty in girls with Williams syndrome. J Pediatr 2002;141:441–444.
57 Douchi T, Maruta K, Kuwahata R, Nagata Y: Precocious puberty in a Williams syndrome patient. Obstet Gynecol 1999;94:860.
58 Virdis R, Street ME, Zampolli M, Radetti G, Pezzini B, Benelli M, et al: Precocious puberty in girls adopted from developing countries. Arch Dis Child 1998;78:152–154.
59 Bourguignon JP, Gerard A, Alvarez Gonzalez ML, Fawe L, Franchimont P: Effects of changes in nutritional conditions on timing of puberty: Clinical evidence from adopted children and experimental studies in the male rat. Horm Res 1992;38:97–105.
60 Mul D, Oostdijk W, Drop SL: Early puberty in adopted children. Horm Res 2002;57:1–9.
61 Parent AS, Teilmann G, Juul A, Skakkebaek NE, Toppari J, Bourguignon JP: The timing of normal puberty and the age limits of sexual precocity: Variations around the world, secular trends, and changes after migration. Endocr Rev 2003;24:668–693.
62 Bona G, Marinello D: Precocious puberty in immigrant children: Indications for treatment. J Pediatr Endocrinol Metab 2000;13(suppl 1):831–834.
63 Teilmann G, Juul A, Skakkebaek NE, Toppari J: Putative effects of endocrine disrupters on pubertal development in the human. Best Pract Res Clin Endocrinol Metab 2002;16:105–121.
64 Krstevska-Konstantinova M, Charlier C, Craen M, Du CM, Heinrichs C, de Beaufort C, et al: Sexual precocity after immigration from developing countries to Belgium: Evidence of previous exposure to organochlorine pesticides. Hum Reprod 2001;16:1020–1026.
65 Dacou-Voutetakis C, Karidis N: Congenital adrenal hyperplasia complicated by central precocious puberty: Treatment with LHRH-agonist analogue. Ann NY Acad Sci 1993;687:250–254.
66 Frenzel S, Doerr HG: Problems of delayed diagnosis of an uncomplicated adrenogenital syndrome (AGS) with 21-hydroxylase defect in a 7-year-old boy. Dtsch Med Wochenschr 1998;123: 831–877.
67 Penny R, Olambiwonnu NO, Frasier DS: Precocious puberty following treatment in a 6-year-old male with congenital adrenal hyperplasia: Studies of serum luteinizing hormone (LH), serum follicle stimulating hormone (FSH) and plasma testosterone. J Clin Endocrinol Metab 1973; 36:920–924.
68 Soliman AT, AlLamki M, AlSalmi I, Asfour M: Congenital adrenal hyperplasia complicated by central precocious puberty: Linear growth during infancy and treatment with gonadotropin-releasing hormone analog. Metabolism 1997;46:513–517.
69 Pescovitz OH, Hench K, Green O, Comite F, Loriaux DL, Cutler GB Jr: Central precocious puberty complicating a virilizing adrenal tumor: Treatment with a long-acting LHRH analog. J Pediatr 1985;106:612–614.

70 Rashaud A, Najafizadeh M: True precocious puberty following removal of virilizing adrenal tumor. Int J Endocrinol Metab 2003;2:97–100.
71 Sandrini R, Ribeiro RC, DeLacerda L: Childhood adrenocortical tumors. J Clin Endocrinol Metab 1997;82:2027–2031.
72 Laue L, Jones J, Barnes KM, Cutler GB Jr: Treatment of familial male precocious puberty with spironolactone, testolactone, and deslorelin. J Clin Endocrinol Metab 1993;76:151–155.
73 Laue L, Kenigsberg D, Pescovitz OH, Hench K, Barnes KM, Loriaux DL, et al: Treatment of familial male precocious puberty with spironolactone and testolactone. N Engl J Med 1989;320:196–502.
74 Wu SM, Leschek EW, Brain C, Chan WY: A novel luteinizing hormone receptor mutation in a patient with familial male-limited precocious puberty: Effect of the size of a critical amino acid on receptor activity. Mol Genet Metab 1999;66:68–73.
75 Leschek EW, Cutler GB Jr: Familial male precocious puberty. Curr Ther Endocrinol Metab 1997;6:343–345.
76 Gromoll J, Partsch CJ, Simoni M, Nordhoff V, Sippell WG, Nieschlag E, et al: A mutation in the first transmembrane domain of the lutropin receptor causes male precocious puberty. J Clin Endocrinol Metab 1998;83:476–480.
77 Eugster EA, Rubin SD, Reiter EO, Plourde P, Jou HC, Pescovitz OH, et al: Tamoxifen treatment for precocious puberty in McCune-Albright syndrome: A multicenter trial. J Pediatr 2003;143:60–66.
78 Schmidt H, Kiess W: Secondary central precocious puberty in a girl with McCune-Albright syndrome responds to treatment with GnRH analogue. J Pediatr Endocrinol Metab 1998;11:77–81.
79 Ojeda SR, Urbanski HF: Puberty in the rat; in Knobil E, Neill JD (eds): The Physiology of Reproduction, ed 2. New York, Raven Press, 1994, vol 2, pp 363–409.
80 Ojeda SR, Bilger M: Neuroendocrine regulation of puberty; in Conn PM, Freeman M (eds): Neuroendocrinology in Physiology and Medicine. Totowa, Humana Press, 1999, pp 197–224.
81 DeFazio RA, Heger S, Ojeda SR, Moenter SM: Activation of A-type gamma-aminobutyric acid receptors excites gonadotropin-releasing hormone neurons. Mol Endocrinol 2002;16:2872–2891.
82 Heger S, Bless E, Seney M, Schwarting GA, Bilger M, Mungenast A, et al: Overexpression of glutamic acid decarboxylase-67 (GAD-67) in GnRH neurons disrupts migratory fate and female reproductive function in mice. Endocrinology 2003;in press.
83 Heger S, Jung H, Cabrera R, Mungenast A, Plant T, Kimura S, et al: Global gene expression profiling of the developing primate hypothalamus identifies genes potentially involved in the transcriptional control of puberty. Annual Endocrine Society Meeting, Philadelphia, 2003.
84 Ojeda SR, Heger S: New thoughts on female precocious puberty. J Pediatr Endocrinol Metab 2001;14(3):245–256.
85 Ojeda SR, Prevot V, Heger S: Regulation of puberty. Curr Opin Endocrinol Diab 2001;8:154–160.
86 Ojeda SR, Terasawa E: Neuroendocrine regulation of puberty; in Pfaff D, Arnold A, Etgen A, Fahrbach S, Moss R, Rubin R (eds): Hormones, Brain and Behavior. San Diego, Academic Press, 2002, pp 589–659.
87 Prevot V, Rio C, Cho GJ, Lomniczi A, Heger S, Neville CM, et al: Normal female sexual development requires neuregulin-erbB receptor signaling in hypothalamic astrocytes. J Neurosci 2003;23: 230–239.
88 Prevot V, Rio C, Cho GJ, Ma YJ, Heger S, Ojeda SR, et al: Single astroglial gene defect delays female sexual development. Proc 83rd Ann Meet Endocrine Soc 2001, p 106.
89 Palmert MR, Malin HV, Boepple PA: Unsustained or slowly progressive puberty in young girls: Initial presentation and long-term follow-up of 20 untreated patients. J Clin Endocrinol Metab 1999;84:415–423.
90 Partsch CJ, Hümmelink R, Lorenzen F, Sippell WG: The significance and characteristics of the LHRH test in diagnosing precocious puberty development in girls: The stimulated LH/FSH quotient differentiates between central precocious puberty and premature thelarche. Monatsschr Kinderheilkd 1989;137:284–288.
91 Heger S, Partsch CJ, Sippell WG: Long-term outcome after depot gonadotropin-releasing hormone agonist treatment of central precocious puberty: Final height, body proportions, body composition, bone mineral density, and reproductive function. J Clin Endocrinol Metab 1999;84:4583–4590.
92 Partsch CJ, Sippell WG: Treatment of central precocious puberty. Best Pract Res Clin Endocrinol Metab 2002;16:165–189.

93 Boyar RM, Finkelstein JW, David R, Roffwarg H, Kapen S, Weitzman ED, et al: Twenty-four hour patterns of plasma luteinizing hormone and follicle-stimulating hormone in sexual precocity. N Engl J Med 1973;289:282–286.
94 Cavallo A, Richards GE, Busey S, Michaels SE: A simplified gonadotrophin-releasing hormone test for precocious puberty. Clin Endocrinol 1995;42:641–646.
95 Muller J, Juul A, Andersson AM, Sehested A, Skakkebaek NE: Hormonal changes during GnRH analogue therapy in children with central precocious puberty. J Pediatr Endocrinol Metab 2000;13:739–746.
96 Chalumeau M, Hadjiathanasiou CG, Ng SM, Cassio A, Mul D, Cisternino M, et al: Selecting girls with precocious puberty for brain imaging: Validation of European evidence-based diagnosis rule. J Pediatr 2003;143:445–450.
97 Cacciari E, Zucchini S, Carla G, Pirazzoli P, Cicognani A, Mandini M, et al: Endocrine function and morphological findings in patients with disorders of the hypothalamic-pituitary area: a study with magnetic resonance. Arch Dis Child 1990;65:1199–1202.
98 Robben SGF, Oostdijk W, Drop SL, Tanghe HL, Vielvoye GJ, Meradji M: Idiopathic isosexual central precocious puberty: Magnetic resonance findings in 30 patients. Brit J Radiol 1995;68:34–38.
99 Chemaitilly W, Trivin C, Adan L, Gall V, Sainte-Rose C, Brauner R: Central precocious puberty: Clinical and laboratory features. Clin Endocrinol (Oxf) 2001;54:289–294.
100 Bridges NA, Cooke A, Healy MJ, Hindmarsh PC, Brook CG: Standards for ovarian volume in childhood and puberty. Fertil Steril 1993;60:456–460.
101 Salardi S, Orsini LF, Cacciari E, Bovicelli L, Tassoni P, Reggiani A: Pelvic ultrasonography in premenarcheal girls: Relation to puberty and sex hormone concentrations. Arch Dis Child 1985;60: 120–125.
102 Salardi S, Orsini LF, Cacciari E, Partesotti S, Brondelli L, Cicognani A, et al: Pelvic ultrasonography in girls with precocious puberty, congenital adrenal hyperplasia, obesity, or hirsutism. J Pediatr 1988;112:880–887.
103 Bridges NA, Cooke A, Healy MJ, Hindmarsh PC, Brook CG: Ovaries in sexual precocity. Clin Endocrinol 1995;42:135–140.
104 Ambrosino MM, Hernanz-Schulman M, Genieser NB, Sklar CA, Fefferman NR, David R: Monitoring of girls undergoing medical therapy for isosexual precocious puberty. J Ultrasound Med 1994;13:501–508.
105 Bridges NA, Cooke A, Healy MJ, Hindmarsh PC, Brook CG: Growth of the uterus. Arch Dis Child 1996;75:330–331.
106 Cassio A, Cacciari E, Zucchini S, Balsamo A, Diegoli M, Orsini LF: Central precocious puberty: Clinical and imaging aspects. J Pediatr Endocrinol Metab 2000;13:703–708.
107 Griffin IJ, Cole TJ, Duncan KA, Hollman AS, Donaldson MD: Pelvic ultrasound findings in different forms of sexual precocity. Acta Paediatr 1995;84:549–554.
108 Kaplan SL, Grumbach MM: Clinical review 14: Pathophysiology and treatment of sexual precocity. J Clin Endocrinol Metab 1990;71:785–789.
109 Léger J, Reynaud R, Czernichow P: Do all girls with apparent idiopathic precocious puberty require gonadotropin-releasing hormone agonist treatment? J Pediatr 2000;137:819–825.
110 Oerter-Klein K: Precocious puberty: Who has it? Who should be treated? J Clin Endocrinol Metab 1999;84:411–414.
111 Rosenfield RL: Selection of children with precocious puberty for treatment with gonadotropin releasing hormone analogs. J Pediatr 1994;124:989–991.
112 Ritzen EM: Early puberty: What is normal and when is treatment indicated? Horm Res 2003;60: 31–34.
113 Mul D, Versluis-den Bieman HJ, Slijper FM, Oostdijk W, Waelkens JJ, Drop SL: Psychological assessments before and after treatment of early puberty in adopted children. Acta Paediatr 2001; 80:965–971.
114 Stattin H: Adult outcome of early puberty in girls. Ped Res 2001;49:6.
115 O'Sullivan E, O'Sullivan M: Precocious puberty: A parent's perspective. Arch Dis Child 2002;86: 320–321.
116 Hamilton AS, Mack TM: Puberty and genetic susceptibility to breast cancer in a case-control study in twins. N Engl J Med 2003;348:2313–2322.

117 Reiter EO, Kaplan SL, Conte FA, Grumbach MM: Responsivity of pituitary gonadotropes to luteinizing hormone-releasing factor in idiopathic precocious puberty, precocious thelarche, precocious adrenarche, and in patients treated with medroxyprogesterone acetate. Pediatr Res 1975;9:111–116.
118 Stanhope R, Pringle PJ, Adams J, Jeffcoate SL, Brook CG: Spontaneous gonadotrophin pulsatility and ovarian morphology in girls with central precocious puberty treated with cyproterone acetate. Clin Endocrinol (Oxf) 1985;23:547–553.
119 Werder EA, Murset G, Zachmann M, Brook CG, Prader A: Treatment of precocious puberty with cyproterone acetate. Pediatr Res 1974;8:248–256.
120 Sadeghi-Nejad A, Kaplan SL, Grumbach MM: The effect of medroxyprogesterone acetate on adrenocortical function in children with precocious puberty. J Pediatr 1971;78:616–624.
121 Cornea A, Janovick JA, Maya-Nunez G, Conn PM: Gonadotropin-releasing hormone receptor microaggregation. Rate monitored by fluorescence resonance energy transfer. J Biol Chem 2001;276:2153–2158.
122 Conn PM, Janovick JA, Stanislaus D, Kuphal D, Jennes L: Molecular and cellular bases of gonadotropin-releasing hormone action in the pituitary and central nervous system. Vitam Horm 1995;50:151–214.
123 Conn PM, Crowley WFJ: Gonadotropin-releasing hormone and its analogs. Annu Rev Med 1994;45:391–405.
124 Lahlou N, Carel JC, Chaussain JL, Roger M: Pharmacokinetics and pharmacodynamics of GnRH agonists: Clinical implications in pediatrics. J Pediatr Endocrinol Metab 2000;13(suppl 1):723–737.
125 Comite F, Cutler GB Jr, Rivier J, Vale W, Loriaux DL, Crowley WFJ: Short-term treatment of idiopathic precocious puberty with a long-acting analogue of luteinizing hormone-releasing hormone. N Engl J Med 1981;305:1546–1550.
126 Laron Z, Kauli R, Ben Zeev Z, Comaru-Schally Am, Schally AV: D-Trp^{6}-analogue of luteinising hormone releasing hormone in combination with cyproterone acetate to treat precocious puberty. Lancet 1981;ii:959–988.
127 Partsch CJ, Hümmelink R, Peter M, Sippell WG, Oostdijk W, Odink RJ, et al: Comparison of complete and incomplete suppression of pituitary-gonadal activity in girls with central precocious puberty: Influence on growth and predicted final height. The German-Dutch Precocious Puberty Study Group. Horm Res 1993;39:111–117.
128 Antoniazzi F, Cisternino M, Nizzoli G, Bozzola M, Corrias A, De Luca F, et al: Final height in girls with central precocious puberty: Comparison of two different luteinizing hormone-releasing hormone agonist treatments. Acta Paediatr 1994;83:1052–1056.
129 Tuvemo T, Gustafsson J, Proos LA, Swedish Growth Hormone Group: Suppression of puberty in girls with short-acting intranasal versus subcutaneous depot GnRH agonist. Horm Res 2002;57:27–31.
130 Bouvattier C, Coste J, Rodrique D, Teinturier C, Carel JC, Chaussain JL, et al: Lack of effect of GnRH agonists on final height in girls with advanced puberty: A randomized long-term pilot study. J Clin Endocrinol Metab 1999;84:3575–3578.
131 Oostdijk W, Hümmelink R, Odink RJ, Partsch CJ, Drop SL, Lorenzen F, et al: Treatment of children with central precocious puberty by a slow-release GnRH agonist. Eur J Pediatr 1990;149:308–313.
132 Carel JC, Lahlou N, Guazzarotti L, Joubert-Collin M, Roger M, Colle M, et al: Treatment of central precocious puberty with depot leuprorelin. French Leuprorelin Trial Group. Eur J Endocrinol 1995;132:699–704.
133 Neely EK, Hintz RL, Parker B, Bachrach LK, Cohen P, Olney R, et al: Two-year results of treatment with depot leuprolide acetate for central precocious puberty. J Pediatr 1992;121:634–640.
134 Parker KL, Baens-Bailon RG, Lee PA: Depot leuprolide acetate dosage for sexual precocity. J Clin Endocrinol Metab 1991;73:50–52.
135 Partsch CJ, Peter M, Brand M, Sippell WG: Treatment of progressive central precocious puberty with leuprorelin depot. Monatsschr Kinderheilkd 1999;147:638–647.
136 Partsch CJ, von Buren E, Brand M, Heger S, Sippell WG: Efficacy of the subcutaneous reformulated triptorelin depot in children with central precocious puberty. Acta Paediatr 1998;87:1240–1244.
137 Oostdijk W, Rikken B, Schreuder S, Otten BJ, Odink RJ, Rouwe C, et al: Final height in central precocious puberty after long term treatment with a slow release GnRH agonist. Arch Dis Child 1996;75:292–297.

138 Tanaka T, Hibi I, Kato K, Saito S, Shimizu N, Suwa S, et al: A dose finding study of a super long-acting luteinizing hormone-releasing hormone analog (leuprolide acetate depot, TAP-144-SR) in the treatment of precocious puberty. Endocrinol Jpn 1991;38:369–376.
139 Okada H: One- and three-month release injectable microspheres of the LH-RH superagonist leuprorelin acetate. Adv Drug Deliv Rev 1997;28:43–70.
140 Lee M, Browneller R, Wu Z, Jung A, Ratanawong C, Sharifi R: Therapeutic effects of leuprorelin microspheres in prostate cancer. Adv Drug Deliv Rev 1997;28:121–138.
141 Carel JC, Lahlou N, Jaramillo O, Montauban V, Teinturier C, Colle M, et al: Treatment of central precocious puberty by subcutaneous injections of leuprorelin 3-month depot (11.25 mg). J Clin Endocrinol Metab 2002;87:4111–4116.
142 Schroeter M, Baus I, Sippell WG, Partsch CJ: Long-term suppression of pituitary-gonadal function with three-month depot of leuprorelin acetate in a girl with central precocious puberty. Horm Res 2002;58:292–296.
143 Huirne JA, Lambalk CB: Gonadotropin-releasing-hormone-receptor antagonists. Lancet 2001;358:1793–1803.
144 Partsch CJ, Weinbauer GF, Schlatt S, Sippell WG, Nieschlag E, Schaub J: GnRH agonist and GnRH antagonist for the suppression of puberty in a non-human primate (*Macaca fascicularis*). Eur J Paediatr 1996;155:157.
145 Roth C, Hegemann F, Hildebrandt J, Balzer I, Witt A, Wuttke W, et al: Pituitary and gonadal effects of GnRH (gonadotropin releasing hormone) analogues in two peripubertal female rat models. Pediatr Res 2004;55:126–133.
146 Cassio A, Cacciari E, Balsamo A, Bal M, Tassinari D: Randomised trial of LHRH analogue treatment on final height in girls with onset of puberty aged 7.5–8.5 years. Arch Dis Child 1999;81:329–332.
147 Yanovski JA, Rose SR, Municchi G, Pescovitz OH, Hill SC, Cassorla FG, et al: Treatment with a luteinizing hormone-releasing hormone agonist in adolescents with short stature. N Engl J Med 2003;348:908–917.
148 Mul D, Oostdijk W, Waelkens JJ, Schulpen TW, Drop SL: Gonadotrophin releasing hormone agonist treatment with or without recombinant human GH in adopted children with early puberty. Clin Endocrinol (Oxf) 2001;55:121–129.
149 Tato L, Saggese G, Cavallo A, Antoniazzi F, Corrias A, Pasquino AM, et al: Use of combined Gn-RH agonist and hGH therapy for better attaining the goals in precocious puberty treatment. Horm Res 1995;44:49–54.
150 Tuvemo T, Gustafsson J, Proos LA: Growth hormone treatment during suppression of early puberty in adopted girls. Swedish Growth Hormone Advisory Group. Acta Paediatr 1999;88:928–932.
151 Antoniazzi F, Zamboni G, Bertoldo F, Lauriola S, Mengarda F, Pietrobelli A, et al: Bone mass at final height in precocious puberty after gonadotropin-releasing hormone agonist with and without calcium supplementation. J Clin Endocrinol Metab 2003;88:1096–1101.
152 Kempers MJ, Otten BJ: Idiopathic precocious puberty versus puberty in adopted children; auxological response to gonadotrophin-releasing hormone agonist treatment and final height. Eur J Endocrinol 2002;147:609–616.
153 Salerno M, Di Maio S, Gasparini N, Mariano A, Macchia V, Tenore A: Central precocious puberty: A single blood sample after gonadotropin-releasing hormone agonist administration in monitoring treatment. Horm Res 1998;50:205–211.
154 Kappy MS, Stuart T, Perelman A, Clemons R: Suppression of gonadotropin secretion by a long-acting gonadotropin-releasing hormone analog (leuprolide acetate, Lupron Depot) in children with precocious puberty. J Clin Endocrinol Metab 1989;69:1087–1089.
155 Yeshaya A, Kauschansky A, Orvieto R, Nussinovitch M, Ben-Rafael Z: Prolonged vaginal bleeding during central precocious puberty therapy with a long-acting gonadotropin-releasing hormone agonist. Acta Obstet Gynec Scand 1998;77:327–329.
156 Manasco PK, Pescovitz OH, Blizzard RM: Local reactions to depot leuprolide therapy for central precocious puberty. J Pediatr 1993;123:334–335.
157 Tonini G, Marinoni S, Forelo V, Rustico M: Local reactions to luteinizing hormone releasing hormone analog therapy. J Pediatr 1995;126:159–160.
158 Tonini G, Lazzerini M: Side effects of GnRH analogue treatment in childhood. J Pediatr Endocrinol Metab 2000;13:795–803.

159 Warnock JK, Bundren JC, Morris DW:. Depressive symptoms associated with gonadotropin-releasing hormone agonists. Depression Anxiety 1998;7:171–177.
160 Feuillan PP, Jones J, Barnes KM, Oerter-Klein K, Cutler GB Jr: Reproductive axis after discontinuation of gonadotropin-releasing hormone analog treatment of girls with precocious puberty: Long term follow-up comparing girls with hypothalamic hamartoma to those with idiopathic precocious puberty. J Clin Endocrinol Metab 1999;84:44–49.
161 Palmert MR, Mansfield MJ, Crowley WFJ, Crigler FJ Jr, Crawford JD, Boepple PA: Is obesity an outcome of gonadotropin-releasing hormone agonist administration? Analysis of growth and body composition in 110 patients with central precocious puberty. J Clin Endocrinol Metab 1999;84:4480–4488.
162 Partsch CJ, Heger S, Brand M, Sippell WG: Adipositas bei Mädchen mit Pubertas praecox unter oder nach Therapie mit GnRH-Agonisten (abstract)? Monatsschr Kinderheilkd 1999;147:143.
163 Styne DM, Harris DA, Egli CA, Conte FA, Kaplan SL, Rivier J, et al: Treatment of true precocious puberty with a potent luteinizing hormone-releasing factor agonist: Effect on growth, sexual maturation, pelvic sonography, and the hypothalamic-pituitary-gonadal axis. J Clin Endocrinol Metab 1985;61:142–151.
164 Kreiter ML, Cara JF, Rosenfield RL: Modifying the outcome of complete precocious puberty. To treat or not to treat; in Grave GD, Cutler GB Jr (eds): Sexual Precocity: Etiology, Diagnosis, and Management. New York, Raven Press, 1993, pp 109–120.
165 Lee PA: Laboratory monitoring of children with precocious puberty. Arch Pediatr Adolesc Med 1994;148:369–376.
166 Lawson ML, Cohen N: A single sample subcutaneous luteinizing hormone (LH)-releasing hormone (LHRH) stimulation test for monitoring LH suppression in children with central precocious puberty receiving LHRH agonists. J Clin Endocrinol Metab 1999;84:4536–4540.
167 Mul D, de Muinck Keizer-Schrama SMPF, Oostdijk W, Drop SL: Auxological and biochemical evaluation of pubertal suppression with the GnRH agonist leuprolide acetate in early and precocious puberty. Horm Res 1999;51:270–276.
168 Maesaka H, Suwa S, Tachibana K, Kikuchi N: Monthly urinary LH and FSH secretory patterns in normal children and patients with sexual disorders. Pediatr Res 1990;28:405–410.
169 Witchel SF, Baens-Bailon RG, Lee PA: Treatment of central precocious puberty: Comparison of urinary gonadotropin excretion and gonadotropin-releasing hormone (GnRH) stimulation tests in monitoring GnRH analog therapy. J Clin Endocrinol Metab 1996;81:1353–1356.
170 Jensen AM, Brocks V, Holm K, Laursen EM, Mueller J: Central precocious puberty in girls: Internal genitalia before, during, and after treatment with long-acting gonadotropin-releasing hormone analogues. J Pediatr 1998;132:105–108.
171 Andolf E: Pelvic ultrasonography cannot alone be used to diagnose pubertal anomalies. Acta Paediatr 2004;88:246–247.
172 Jay N, Mansfield MJ, Bizz, Blizzard RM, Crowley WFJ, Schoenfeld D, et al: Ovulation and menstrual function of adolescent girls with central precocious puberty after therapy with gonadotropin-releasing hormone agonists. J Clin Endocrinol Metab 1992;75:890–894.
173 Schroor EJ, van Weissenbruch MM, Delemarre-van de Waal HA: Long-term GnRH-agonist treatment does not postpone central development of the GnRH pulse generator in girls with idiopathic precocious puberty. J Clin Endocrinol Metab 1995;80:1696–1701.
174 Boepple PA, Mansfield MJ, Crawford JD, Crigler FJ Jr, Blizzard RM, Crowley WFJ: Completion of growth and puberty in girls with central precocious puberty following long-term GnRH agonist-induced pituitary-gonadal suppression; in Plant T, Lee PA (eds): The Neurobiology of Puberty. Bristol, Journal of Endocrinology, 1995, pp 327–334.
175 Lazar L, Kauli R, Pertzelan A, Phillip M: Gonadotropin-suppressive therapy in girls with early and fast puberty affects the pace of puberty but not total pubertal growth or final height. J Clin Endocrinol Metab 2002;87:2090–2094.
176 Wacharasindhu S, Srivuthana S, Aroonparkmongkol S, Supornsilchai V, Hiranrat P, Yodvisitsak V: Final adult height in 'early normal pubertal girls' treated with gonadotropin releasing hormone agonists. J Med Assoc Thai 2003;86(suppl 2):S170–S173.
177 Bayley N, Pinneau SR: Tables for predicting adult height from skeletal age: Revised use with the Greulich-Pyle hand standards. J Pediatr 1952;40:423–441.

178 Greulich W, Pyle S: Radiographic Atlas of Skeletal Development of the Hand and Wrist. Stanford, Stanford University Press, 1959.
179 Tanner JM, Whitehoure RH, Cameron N, Marshall WA, Healy MJ, Goldstein H: Assessment of Skeletal Maturity and Prediction of Adult Height (TW2 Method), ed 2. London, Academic Press, 1983.
180 Bar A, Linder B, Sobel EH, Saenger P, DiMartino-Nardi J: Bayley-Pinneau method of height prediction in girls with central precocious puberty: Correlation with adult height. J Pediatr 1995;126:955–958.
181 Kauli R, Galatzer a, Kornreich L, Lazar L, Pertzelan A, Laron Z: Final height of girls with central precocious puberty, untreated versus treated with cyproterone acetate or GnRH analogue. A comparative study with re-evaluation of predictions by the Bayley-Pinneau method. Horm Res 1997; 47:54–61.
182 Lazar L, Pertzelan A, Weintrob N, Philipp M, Kauli R: Sexual precocity in boys: Accelerated versus slowly progressive puberty gonadotropin-suppressive therapy and final height. J Clin Endocrinol Metab 2001;86:4127–4132.
183 Oerter KE, Manasco PK, Barnes KM, Jones J, Hill SC, Cutler GB Jr: Adult height in precocious puberty after long-term treatment with deslorelin. J Clin Endocrinol Metab 1991;73: 1235–1240.
184 Antoniazzi F, Arrigo T, Cisternino M, Galluzzi F, Bertelloni S, Pasquino AM, et al: End results in central precocious puberty with GnRH analog treatment: The data of the Italian Study Group for Physiopathology of Puberty. J Pediatr Endocrinol Metab 2000;13:773–780.
185 Arrigo T, Cisternino M, Galluzzi F, Bertelloni S, Pasquino AM, Antoniazzi F, et al: Analysis of the factors affecting auxological response to GnRH agonist treatment and final height outcome in girls with idiopathic central precocious puberty. Eur J Endocrinol 1999;141:140–144.
186 Partsch CJ, Heger S, Sippell WG: Treatment of central precocious puberty: Lessons from a 15 years prospective trial. German Decapeptyl Study Group. J Pediatr Endocrinol Metab 2000;13 (suppl 1):747–758.
187 Antoniazzi F, Bertoldo F, Zamboni G, Valentini R, Sirpresi S, Cavallo L, et al: Bone mineral metabolism in girls with precocious puberty during gonadotrophin-releasing hormone agonist treatment. Eur J Endocrinol 1995;133:412–417.
188 Bertelloni S, Baroncelli GI, Sorrentino MC, Perri G, Saggese G: Effect of central precocious puberty and gonadotropin-releasing hormone analogue treatment on peak bone mass and final height in females. Eur J Pediatr 1998;157:363–367.
189 Boot AM, de Muinck Keizer-Schrama SMPF, Pols HA, Krenning EP, Drop SL: Bone mineral density and body composition before and during treatment with gonadotropin-releasing hormone agonist in children with central precocious and early puberty. J Clin Endocrinol Metab 1998;83:370–373.
190 Unal O, Berberoglu M, Evliyaoglu O, Adiyaman P, Aycan Z, Ocal G: Effects on bone mineral density of gonadotropin releasing hormone analogs used in the treatment of central precocious puberty. J Pediatr Endocrinol Metab 2003;16:407–411.
191 Baumann DA, Landolt MA, Wetterwald R, Dubuis JM, Sizonenko PC, Werder EA: Psychological evaluation of young women after medical treatment for central precocious puberty. Horm Res 2001;56:45–50.
192 Schoevaart CE, Drop SL, Otten BJ, Slijper FM, Degenhart HJ: Growth analysis up to final height and psychosocial adjustment of treated and untreated patients with precocious puberty. Horm Res 1990;34:197–203.
193 Lee PA: Medroxyprogesterone therapy for sexual precocity in girls. Am J Dis Child 1981;135: 443–445.
194 Brauner R, Adan L, Malandry F, Zantleifer D: Adult height in girls with idiopathic true precocious puberty. J Clin Endocrinol Metab 1994;79:415–420.
195 Stasiowska B, Vannelli S, Benso L: Final height in sexually precocious girls after therapy with an intranasal analogue of gonadotrophin-releasing hormone (buserelin). Horm Res 1994;42:81–85.
196 Paul D, Conte FA, Grumbach MM, Kaplan SL: Long-term effect of gonadotropin-releasing hormone agonist therapy on final and near-final height in 26 children with true precocious puberty treated at a median age of less than 5 years. J Clin Endocrinol Metab 1995;80:546–551.

197 Kato K, Fujimoto M, Hibi I, Suwa S, Shimizu N: The long-term effect of cyproterone acetate on growth in girls with idiopathic precocious puberty. Androcur Study Group in Japan. Eur J Pediatr 1993;152:297–300.
198 Boepple PA, Crowley WF Jr: Gonadotrophin-releasing hormone analogues as therapeutic probes in human growth and development: Evidence from children with central precocious puberty. Acta Paediatr Scand Suppl 1991;372:33–38.
199 Cacciari E, Cassio A, Balsamo A, Colli C, Cicognani A, Pirazzoli P, et al: Long-term follow-up and final height in girls with central precocious puberty treated with luteinizing hormone-releasing hormone analogue nasal spray. Arch Pediatr Adolesc Med 1994;148:1194–1199.
200 Klein KO, Barnes KM, Jones JV, Feuillan PP, Cutler GB Jr: Increased final height in precocious puberty after long-term treatment with LHRH agonists: The National Institutes of Health experience. J Clin Endocrinol Metab 2001;86:4711–4716.
201 Kauli R, Kornreich L, Laron Z: Pubertal development, growth and final height in girls with sexual precocity after therapy with the GnRH analogue D-TRP-6-LHRH. A report on 15 girls, followed after cessation of gonadotrophin suppressive therapy. Horm Res 1990;33:11–17.
202 Galluzzi F, Salti R, Bindi G, Pasquini E, La Cauza C: Adult height comparison between boys and girls with precocious puberty after long-term gonadotrophin-releasing hormone analogue therapy. Acta Paediatr 1998;87:521–527.
203 Carel JC, Roger M, Ispas S, Tondu F, Lahlou N, Blumberg J, et al: Final height after long-term treatment with triptorelin slow release for central precocious puberty: Importance of statural growth after interruption of treatment. French study group of Decapeptyl in Precocious Puberty. J Clin Endocrinol Metab 1999;84:1973–1978.
204 Mul D, Oostdijk W, Otten BJ, Rouwe C, Jansen M, Delemarre-van de Waal HA, et al: Final height after gonadotrophin releasing hormone agonist treatment for central precocious puberty: The Dutch experience. J Pediatr Endocrinol Metab 2000;13:765–772.
205 Pucarelli I, Segni M, Ortore M, Arcadi E, Pasquino AM: Effects of combined gonadotropin-releasing hormone agonist and growth hormone therapy on adult height in precocious puberty: A further contribution. J Pediatr Endocrinol Metab 2003;16:1005–1010.
206 Rizzo V, De SV, Corrias A, Fortini M, Galluzzi F, Bertelloni S, et al: Factors influencing final/near-final height in 12 boys with central precocious puberty treated with gonadotrophin-releasing hormone agonists. Italian Study Group of Physiopathology of Puberty. J Pediatr Endocrinol Metab 2000;13(suppl 1):781–786.
207 Mul D, Bertelloni S, Carel JC, Saggese G, Chaussain JL, Oostdijk W: Effect of gonadotropin-releasing hormone agonist treatment in boys with central precocious puberty: Final height results. Horm Res 2002;58:1–7.
208 Lanes R, Soros A, Jakubowicz S: Accelerated versus slowly progressive forms of puberty in girls with precocious and early puberty. Gonadotropin suppressive effect and final height obtained with two different analogs. J Pediatr Endocrinol Metab 2004;17:759–766.
209 Paterson WF, McNeill E, Young D, Donaldson MD: Auxological outcome and time to menarche following long-acting goserelin therapy in girls with central precocious or early puberty. Clin Endocrinol 2004;61:626–634.

Priv.-Doz. Dr. med. C.-J. Partsch
Klinik für Kinder und Jugendliche, Städtische Kliniken
Hirschlandstrasse 97, Esslingen D–73730 (Germany)
Tel. +49 711 3103 35 00, Fax +49 711 3103 35 25, E-Mail j.partsch@kliniken-es.de

Delemarre-van de Waal HA (ed): Abnormalities in Puberty. Scientific and Clinical Advances.
Endocr Dev. Basel, Karger, 2005, vol 8, pp 126–136

Very Long-Term Follow-Up of Girls with Early and Late Menarche

Therése Johansson[a], *E. Martin Ritzén*[b]

[a]Department of Behavioural, Social and Legal Sciences, Örebro University, Örebro, and [b]Department of Woman and Child Health, Karolinska Institute, Stockholm, Sweden

Abstract

Short- and long-term psychosocial effects of precocious or early normal puberty are probably more important for individuals than the moderate losses in final height they experience. Despite this, pediatric endocrinologists have focused much more on final height than psychosocial outcomes. As a surrogate for long-term follow-up studies of girls with precocious puberty, we have reviewed the results of a very long-term study of physical and psychosocial development of girls with normal early puberty. Results revealed that at age 15–16, girls with menarche before age 11 (early) were more norm-breaking, including being delinquents. In addition, they had earlier advanced sexual experiences. By adult age, there were no differences in psychosocial adjustment between the early- and late-developed women. Thus, the effects of early pubertal timing for psychosocial problems seem to be adolescent-limited. At ages 27 and 43, early-developed women had lower academic education. Regarding somatic development, at age 43, women with early menarche were shorter and heavier, had worse physical fitness and dieted more frequently compared to other women. There was no difference in quality of life. In searching for reasons for the antisocial behaviors in adolescence and the lower educational levels among early developers, early heterosexual relations seem to be the most crucial.

Early pubertal development in girls is one of the most frequent causes of referral to pediatric endocrinology clinics. Some girls may be classified as true precocious puberty (in Caucasians two signs of puberty before age 8 years), but worries are frequent even if the pubertal development can be regarded as 'early normal'. In most cases, there is no pathology to be found even after extensive work-up. Still, both parents and referring physicians may be worried about the early development, and questions about possible long term somatic and psychosocial consequences of the early maturation are common. To answer these questions, the pediatric endocrinologist needs to consult publications that describe the natural outcome of precocious puberty and early normal puberty what concerns both soma and psyche. The conclusions are critical, since if the short- or long-term outcome is expected to be disadvantageous, treatment with gonadotropin-releasing hormone superagonists (GnRH agonists) for many years will be considered.

There is an abundant literature on growth of early maturing girls, with and without treatment [1–4]. There is consensus that precocious puberty that starts before age 6 will end up with shorter adult stature than the average girl, and the final height of these early maturers will benefit from long-term GnRH agonist treatment. Even if puberty starts somewhat later (up to 8 years), the girls with a rapid advancement of pubertal signs and advanced bone age will probably also end up taller if treated [5]. It is remarkable that almost all studies have focused on the outcome in centimeters, rather than in quality of life. The latter has been the subject of many studies of short young adults in general, with or without a specific diagnosis, with and without treatment aimed to improve final height. To our knowledge, *none* of these studies has been able to demonstrate that the quality of life is poorer among short adults than among those with average height. Neither has it been shown that adding some centimeters to the final height will significantly increase their quality of life. Therefore, other factors than final height should be considered when the decision to treat or not to treat girls with precocious or early puberty is made.

At the time of consultation, girls with precocious puberty have significantly more concerns over physical differences from peers, and as a group, they are more depressed, moody, withdrawn. Treatment with GnRH agonists reduces concerns, if breasts disappear or regress markedly [6–8] [TJ5]. For some girls this is important and GnRHa treatment is thus indicated. Yet, others may be less worried. The long-term somatic and psychosocial consequences of their early maturation should still be evaluated in order to counsel the girls and the parents in a professionally correct way.

To our knowledge, there are no follow-up studies performed for girls with precocious puberty into adulthood. However, the very long-term studies of girls with early normal puberty [9, Stattin et al., unpubl., Johansson et al., unpubl.] to be reviewed below, in addition to new data on weight, height, dieting behavior, and quality of life presented here, should work as a reasonable surrogate.

Study Population

In 1965, all girls born during the year 1955 in a middle Swedish town of 100,000 inhabitants were invited to participate in a prospective study of growth

Table 1. Number and percentage of girls that reported menarche at the different age groups: mean age of menarche for the whole group was 12.9 years

Age at menarche	n	Percent of total
<11 years ('early')	49	10.5
11–12 years	108	23.2
12–13 years	186	39.9
>13 years ('late')	123	26.4
Total	466	100

and psychosocial development. More than 90% of the girls in the town born in 1955 (466 girls and their families) accepted. Information about a wide variety of psychological and social issues was collected at the age of 10, and participants were then measured and interviewed at 13, 15, 27 and 43 years of age. The participation rate at the latest time of study (1998) was 89%. All studies were approved by the appropriate ethics committees. The subjects of this study have been divided into four menarcheal groups (table 1). First, we present new data on adult height and weight, physical fitness and dieting behavior for girls of the four groups. Next, we will summarize the findings that relate to the role of age of pubertal development (age of menarche) for psychosocial adjustment in adolescence and adulthood. In the final section of this chapter, we discuss lessons to be learned for the management of early puberty in the pediatric endocrine clinic.

Development of Height and Weight

At age 13, there was a negative correlation between height and the age of menarche, as expected (fig. 1), with early-developing girls being taller than other girls were.

The degree of pubertal maturation was also reflected by a greater body mass index (BMI) of the early maturing girls. The difference in height between the early and the late-developed group had reverted to the opposite at age 43, when the early group was 3 cm shorter than the latest group. However, they were 6 kg heavier. Thus, the BMI at age 43 was 3 units higher in the women with early menarche than in those with late menarche (fig. 2). In accordance with their higher BMI scores, compared to late-maturing women, the circumference of early maturers' waistlines and hips were on average 6 cm wider respectively. The differences were significant. However, the waist/hip ratios were not different between the groups.

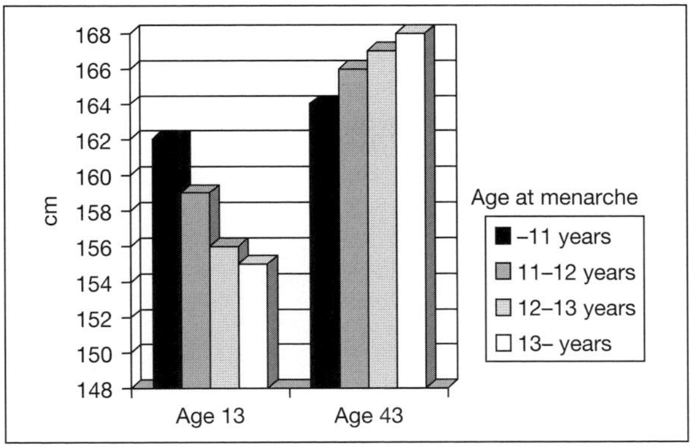

Fig. 1. Height at ages 13 and 43 of the four groups with different age of menarche.

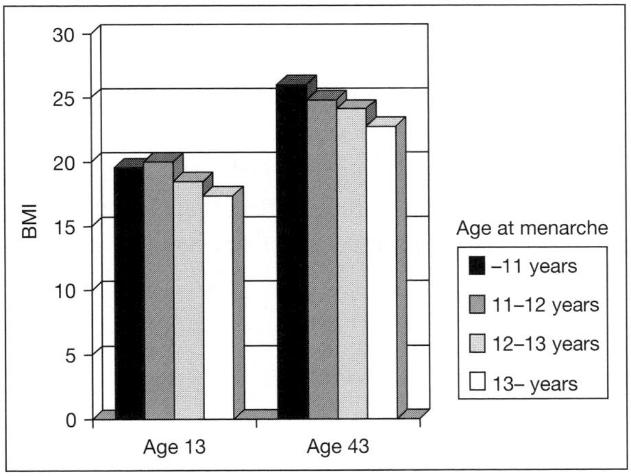

Fig. 2. BMI at ages 13 and 43 for the groups with menarche at the indicated ages.

Physical Fitness

Next, we were interested in physical fitness of the subjects. At age 43, the women graded their physical fitness as their ability to walk, jog or run for 2 km (table 2). They were asked if they agreed to one of the statements shown in table 2.

Figure 3 shows a summary of the answers. The women with early menarche considered themselves less fit ($p < 0.05$) than those with average or late menarche.

Table 2. Questions asked in order to estimate the degree of physical fitness

Statement	Fitness score
I cannot walk 2 km without a rest	1
I can walk 2 km without a rest	2
I can jog 2 km if I stop and rest a couple of times	3
I can jog 2 km without a rest	4
I can run 2 km at a good speed, if I can stop and rest a couple of times	5
I can run 2 km at a good speed without a rest	6
I can run 2 km at high speed without a rest	7

Body Dissatisfaction: Dieting Behavior

At age 43, participants reported on their dieting behaviors. The question was 'How often do you diet?' Answers ranged from (1) No, never, (2) Yes, occasionally, to (3) Yes, often or almost always. The results revealed that women with early menarche were dieting significantly more often than other women did (fig. 4); indicating lower satisfaction with body weight among early maturers compared to other women.

Psychosocial Development

The psychosocial development of the different groups will be published elsewhere [Johansson et al., unpubl. data, Stattin et al., unpubl. data]. A short summary will be given below in addition to new data on the influence of pubertal maturation and height on quality of life in middle adulthood.

The relations between adolescent psychosocial problems and early puberty have been investigated thoroughly. Several reviews [9–13], along with empirical studies on clinical samples [6, 7] have reported that girls with early pubertal timing seem to have more social problems and more internal distress in adolescence than other girls do. The question is if this is a temporary, adolescent phenomenon, or if these problems continue in adulthood.

In agreement with previous research [11, 13], the study summarized here revealed that the mid-adolescent years were problematic in many ways for the early-maturing girls: At age 15–16, those with menarche before age 11 were more delinquent, were more often in conflict with parents and teachers, used

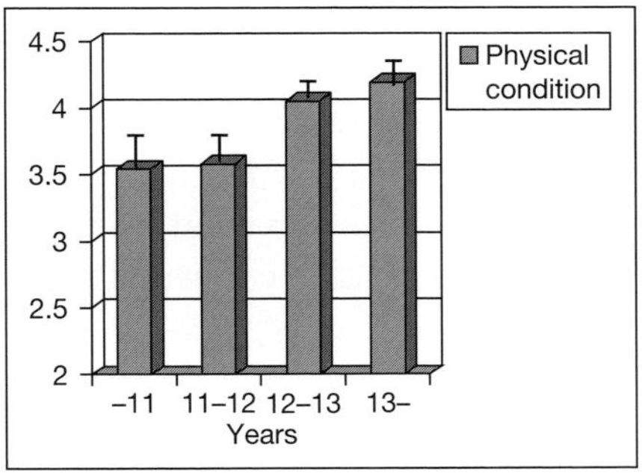

Fig. 3. Physical fitness scores of the groups with different ages of menarche at age 43 years, as evaluated by themselves. The columns represent mean and SE of the scores described in table 2.

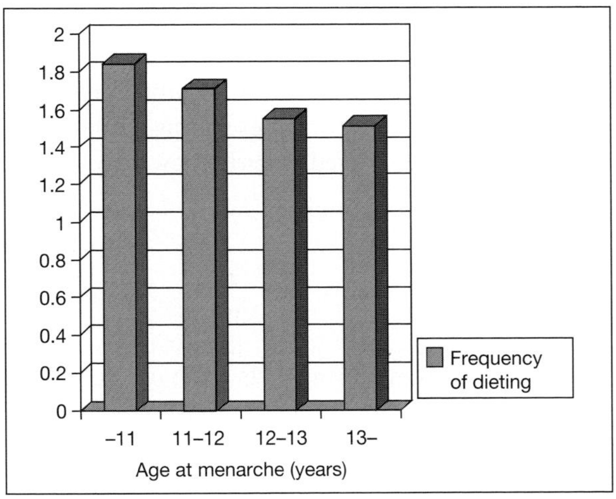

Fig. 4. Frequency of dieting at age 43 for the four groups with different ages at menarche.

more of alcohol and drugs and they had more advanced sexual experiences. They were also more often registered for criminal offences. However, by the age of 27 years, there were no differences between the early and late-developed women with the respect to drinking, criminal offences, or other measures of psychosocial problems. This was also the situation when the subjects were 43 years of age. Thus, the more problematic conduct of the early developers seems to be limited to adolescence.

On the other hand, at the age 27 there were differences in attained education between the four menarcheal groups. First, it should be observed that there were no differences in IQ between the four groups. At the ages of 10 and 13, school performances were equal between the groups. On the other hand, by 15–16 years of age the girls with menarche before age 11 had significantly lower grades and were less motivated for schoolwork. They finished school at an earlier age, and at age 27, they had reached a lower level of academic studies than those with late puberty. By age 43, the early developers had caught up in academic training. Nevertheless, even at this age, fewer women with early menarche had a university education compared to the late developers.

In searching for the reasons for the differences in education between the early and late maturers, one factor dominates: In mid-adolescence, girls with early menarche significantly more often had advanced opposite sex relations, often with an older male. Actually, heterosexual relations was the factor that correlated most strongly with social problem behaviors when the influence of pubertal timing and regular heterosexual relations were compared. Socioeconomic status of the girls' families did not seem to be of important in this regard.

The girls in the original study were born in 1955. The findings reported here for the adolescent years seem to be valid also for present day adolescents, since studies performed in 1998 of 15-year-old Swedish girls show very similar findings [Stattin et al., unpubl. data].

Quality of Life in Adulthood

Several studies have reported that early-maturing girls are more depressed and have worse self-images, particularly body images, than other girls in adolescence [10–12]. Are early maturers likely to be less happy in adulthood as well? We used a battery of instruments to measure life satisfaction and positive self-image at age 43. Positive affect was measured with the scale 'General positive affect' in the Mental Health Inventory [14]. The scale comprises nine questions concerning subjects' feelings of being happy, satisfied, forward looking, relaxed, calm and peaceful, etc., during the past month (alpha = 0.92). Self-image is a scale that measures positive perception of oneself. It contains four questions like 'I am proud of the type of person I have become' (alpha = 0.72). Family satisfaction was tapped by one item asking subjects 'Are you happy with your family life?' Work satisfaction was measured with a scale comprising four items such as 'I am satisfied with my current work position' (alpha = 0.84). Subjects' reported on their leisure satisfaction by answering a single question about how happy they were with their leisure times. Life satisfaction, finally, was assessed using two questions, 'Are you satisfied with your life' and 'How do you like your current life?' The correlation between these two items was 0.35. According to the alpha values, the scales showed satisfying reliabilities overall.

Table 3. Correlations between age at menarche and positive affect, self-image, satisfaction with family, work, leisure and life at age 43

	Age at menarche (n)	Significance	Height (n)	Significance
Positive affect	−0.03 (388)	n.s.	−0.03 (475)	n.s.
Self-image	−0.03 (270)	n.s.	0.04 (298)	n.s.
Family satisfaction	−0.02 (273)	n.s.	−0.07 (300)	n.s.
Work satisfaction	−0.02 (376)	n.s.	0.04 (434)	n.s.
Leisure satisfaction	0.06 (281)	n.s.	−0.08 (308)	n.s.
Life satisfaction	−0.01 (399)	n.s.	0.03 (476)	n.s.

According to the results presented in table 3, there were no significant correlations between pubertal timing and positive affect (i.e. a general feeling of well-being), self-image, or satisfaction in various life domains. Thus, the early-developed women were as happy with themselves and their life as the later-developed women at 43 years of age. Moreover, we correlated height at age 43 with the quality of life measures (table 3). We found no significant correlation between height and quality of life. Women of short stature were equally content with life as tall women were.

Do the Differences between the Early- and the Late-Developed Girls Matter at Age 43?

In the present study, we found that neither pubertal timing nor adult height matters for quality of life in adulthood. Thus, the 3 cm lower adult height of the early girls has little influence on psychological well-being. The higher BMI scores might possibly put them in a higher risk for metabolic problems later in life.

The studies of early maturers' psychosocial development in adolescence are of more concern. The strained relationships with parents and teachers, and their higher frequency of antisocial behaviors at age 15–16 will certainly cause parental distress during adolescence, even if by age 27 everything had 'normalized'. However, some lasting sequelae of their early puberty remained: At the age of 43, the early-developed women perceived themselves to be less physically fit and showed lower body satisfaction. The latter finding is similar to others [15], who have noted that the age of menarche predicts body esteem in midlife. Furthermore, women with early puberty had lower educational levels. Fewer of the early maturing girls had university degrees.

Lessons to be Learned for the Management of Early Puberty in the Pediatric Endocrine Clinic

In the absence of long-term follow-up of girls with precocious puberty, the present and reviewed findings on girls with early normal puberty can serve as a surrogate. The studies summarized showed that the social problems of the early girls were associated with certain types of interpersonal relationships in adolescence. Early pubertal timing was an instigating factor for developing heterosexual relationships early. Early-developed girls with more advanced social relationships, including opposite sex relationships, had more problematic adjustment situations than other girls. The explanation given was that through opposite-sex relations with older males and older peers, early maturing girls encounter peer environments with more advanced social behaviors and are brought into leisure-time settings in which these types of behaviors are more typical. Early-developed girls adjust to the peers that are more advanced, and start to act and behave accordingly. The early developers, who did not establish early opposite sex relations, were not more likely to be problematic in adolescence. The early-maturing girls, who establish heterosexual contacts early in life, seem to lose interest in getting higher education and pursuing academic careers, rather they start having children early. Lower educational attainment was the sole adverse social adult outcome for the early developers with early heterosexual relations.

The obvious message is that parents of early-maturing girls should be informed that girls with early pubertal timing are likely to acquire socially more advanced behaviors at an earlier age. However, in the reviewed studies it is only under conditions that promote access to more advanced peer groups, and particularly opposite-sex relations (often with an older male); that early pubertal timing is linked to problem behavior in adolescence.

It is not known whether the future psychosocial development of early maturing girls will benefit from GnRHa treatment in early pubertal years. The best way of avoiding the problematic situations that early-developed girls will encounter in adolescence and the antisocial behaviors that they might develop is probably through family interaction, or possibly, in some instances, facilitated by GnRH treatment.

Conclusions

Information about natural outcomes of early pubertal maturation is essential to pediatric endocrinologists when counseling early-developed girls and their families. The aim of this chapter was to summarize the findings of a very long-term follow-up of girls with early and late menarche as well as presenting some new related data. At age 43, females with early puberty were shorter and heavier, had worse physical fitness and dieted more frequently compared to women with later age at menarche. The early-developed girls had more psychosocially problematic behaviors at ages 15–16, problems that had disappeared by age 27. Apart from the somatic differences, lower and later achievement of academic training was the only difference that remained at 43 years of age between the menarcheal groups of girls. Regarding quality of life, early-developed females were as happy with themselves, with their works and their families, as later developed females were in midlife. According to the results presented in this chapter, adult height within normal limits does not seem to matter for quality of life.

Acknowledgements

This study was made possible by access to data from the longitudinal research program Individual Development and Adaptation (IDA). The scientific leader is Lars R. Bergman. Responsible for the planning, implementation and financing of the collection of data before 1996 was David Magnusson and after that time Lars R. Bergman. This study was supported by grants from The Bank of Sweden Tercentenary Foundation. We wish to thank Prof. Håkan Stattin for valuable comments on earlier versions of this chapter.

References

1 Heger S, Partsch CJ, Sippell WG: Long-term outcome after depot gonadotropin-releasing hormone agonist treatment of central precocious puberty: Final height, body proportions, body composition, bone mineral density, and reproductive function. J Clin Endocrinol Metab 1999;84:4583–4590.

2 Partsch CJ, Heger S, Sippell WG: Treatment of central precocious puberty: Lessons from a 15 years prospective trial. German Decapeptyl Study Group. J Pediatr Endocrinol Metab 2000;13 (suppl 1):747–758.

3 Mul D, Oostdijk W, Otten BJ, Rouwe C, Jansen M, Delemarre-van de Waal HA, Waelkens JJ, Drop SL: Final height after gonadotropin releasing hormone agonist treatment for central precocious puberty: The Dutch experience. J Pediatr Endocrinol Metab 2000;13(suppl 1):765–772.

4 Klein KO, Barnes KM, Jones JV, Feuillan PP, Cutler GB Jr: Increased final height in precocious puberty after long-term treatment with LHRH agonists: The National Institutes of Health experience. J Clin Endocrinol Metab 2001;86:4711–4716.

5 Ritzén EM: Early puberty: What is normal and when is treatment indicated? Hormone Research 2003;60(suppl 3):31–34.

6 Xhrouet-Heinrichs D, Lagrou K, Heinrichs C, Craen M, Dooms L, Malvaux P, Kanen F, Bourguignon JP: Longitudinal study of behavioral and affective patterns in girls with central precocious puberty during long-acting triptorelin therapy. Acta Paediatr 1997;86:808–815.

7 Mul D, Versluis-den Bieman HJ, Slijper FM, Oostdijk W, Waelkens JJ, Drop SL: Psychological assessments before and after treatment of early puberty in adopted children. Acta Paediatr 2001;90: 965–971.

8 Mul D, Oostdijk W, Waelkens JJ, Schulpen TW, Drop SL: Gonadotrophin releasing hormone agonist treatment with or without recombinant human GH in adopted children with early puberty. Clin Endocrinol (Oxf) 2001;55:121–129.
9 Stattin H, Kerr M, Magnusson D: Psychosocial outcomes of early puberty in females. 6th Joint Meeting of LWPES and ESPE, Montreal, 2001.
10 Alsaker F: The impact of puberty. J Child Psychol Psychiatry 1996;37:249–258.
11 Buchanan CM, Eccles J, Becker JB: Are adolescents the victims of raging hormones? Evidence for activational effects of hormones on moods and behavior in adolescence. Psychol Bull 1992; 111:62–107.
12 Connolly SD, Paikoff RL, Buchanan CM: Puberty: The interplay of biological and psychosocial processes in adolescence; in Adams GR, Montemayor R, Gullotta TP (eds): Psychosocial Development during Adolescence. Thousand Oaks, Sage, 1996, pp 259–299.
13 Stattin H, Magnusson D: Pubertal Maturation in Female Development. Hillsdale, Erlbaum, 1990.
14 Veit CT, Ware JE Jr: The structure of psychological distress and well-being in general populations. J Consult Clin Psychol 1983;51:730–742.
15 McLaren L, Hardy R, Kuh D: Women's body satisfaction at midlife and lifetime body size: A prospective study. Health Psychol 2003;22:370–377.

Therése Johansson, MA
Department of Behavioural, Social and Legal Sciences, Örebro University
Fakultetsgatan 1, SE–701 82 Örebro (Sweden)
Tel. +46 19 301091, Fax +46 19 303484, E-Mail therese.johansson@bsr.oru.se

Delemarre-van de Waal HA (ed): Abnormalities in Puberty. Scientific and Clinical Advances.
Endocr Dev. Basel, Karger, 2005, vol 8, pp 137–149

Polycystic Ovary Syndrome in Adolescence

New Insights in Pathophysiology and Treatment

R. Homburg

Division of Reproductive Medicine, Department of Obstetrics and Gynaecology, Vrije Universiteit Medical Centre, Amsterdam, The Netherlands

Abstract

Polycystic ovary syndrome (PCOS) is a prevalent cause of menstrual disorders, acne and hirsutism presenting during adolescence. In the majority of cases, a familial trait is obvious but the offending genes have yet to be identified. However, much of the pathophysiology of the syndrome causing the overproduction of ovarian androgens is now becoming clearer. The early diagnostic signs are often mistakenly dismissed as 'normal' changes of adolescence but it is important to make an early diagnosis in order to save the adolescent from the early and late stigmata of the syndrome. The avoidance of overweight, frank obesity and the consequential exaggeration of symptoms by the associated insulin resistance is of prime importance as hyperinsulinemia plays a key role in the pathogenesis. Anti-androgens are the most widely used medication and, in combination with estrogen, are capable of restoring menstrual regularity and reducing the symptoms of acne and hirsutism, so important for the improvement of the disturbing psychosocial effect that they may play at this age. The use of metformin, an insulin sensitizer, for affected adolescents is the topic of a presently heated debate.

Introduction

Presenting around the time of the menarche, polycystic ovary syndrome (PCOS) is a very prevalent syndrome in adolescence. Although the pathogenesis of this heterogeneous syndrome is still incompletely determined, the management of the specific symptoms in adult women is now fairly well determined. In adolescents however, the subject of management leaves many questions unanswered.

As some of the accepted symptoms of PCOS (menstrual irregularities, acne) have been associated with a 'normal' adolescence, definitive diagnostic criteria have been blurred. Biochemical features such as increased androgen and insulin secretion, typical of PCOS, are also often a feature of a normal adolescence. Even when the diagnosis of PCOS has been well established, should the condition be managed symptomatically, prophylactically or not at all, at such a young age? These are just some of the questions that the presentation of PCOS in adolescence poses.

Presentation of PCOS in Adolescence

The commonest form of presentation of PCOS in adolescence is persistent menstrual irregularity and/or symptoms of hyperandrogenism. The menstrual irregularities usually consist of oligomenorrhea (>35 days between menstruation) or amenorrhea (>6 months without bleeding). These symptoms reflect ovulatory dysfunction. Oligomenorrhea in adolescents has widely been regarded as a stage in the physiological maturation of the hypothalamic pituitary-ovarian axis. However, today, following close investigation of oligomenorrheic adolescents, it seems that a very large proportion of these have biochemical markers typical of PCOS and eventually develop the further clinical features of the syndrome. For example, 57% of 52 oligomenorrheic 15-year-olds had LH and testosterone levels above the 95th percentile of girls with regular menstrual cycles [1]. Similarly, 32% of adolescents with oligomenorrhea were found to have clinically obvious hirsutism [2] and 21% had acne [3]. If the oligomenorrhea of adolescence does 'correct itself' it is most likely to do so in the first two postmenarchal years. If, after this time, oligomenorrhea persists, it may be regarded as a probable early clinical sign of PCOS and this should be investigated at this stage.

The commonest forms of clinical expression of hyperandrogenism, the fundamental problem in PCOS, are mainly expressed at the level of the skin in the form of hirsutism and acne. Hirsutism is defined as an excess of pigmented, thick terminal hair that appears in a male distribution in androgen sensitive areas. These areas include face, chest, abdomen and thighs. Before puberty, body hair is primarily composed of fine, short, unpigmented villus hairs which during pubarche are stimulated by androgens to become coarse, pigmented, thickened terminal hairs. An excess of androgens will produce such hair growth in a male distribution. Hirsutism may be quantified using the Ferriman-Gallwey score.

Acne vulgaris is a very common condition particularly in adolescents. It is basically caused by increased activity in sebaceous glands which is a manifestation of cutaneous androgenization. It often appears in the teenage years, induced by the burst of pubertal androgenic activity, but if persistent, particularly severe or of late onset, is commonly associated with PCOS.

Although overweight (body mass index, BMI, 26–30) and frank obesity (BMI >30) are not regarded as direct diagnostic signs of PCOS, they are associated with the syndrome in about 40% of adults. Fortunately, they are less common and less pronounced in adolescents but when occurring have a very significant effect on the presenting symptoms.

The typical morphological features of the polycystic ovary can be relatively easily seen on ultrasound examination and their imaging is the single most prevalent diagnostic sign of this heterogeneously presenting syndrome. Biochemical features include raised serum testosterone, androstendione or free androgen index, raised serum LH concentrations and hyperinsulinemia. Similar to the presentation of the symptoms, the biochemical features are inconsistently present, especially when a single blood sample is analyzed and are unnecessary and unreliable for diagnostic purposes.

The earliest recognized sign of PCOS is a premature pubarche. Girls who present in mid-childhood with premature growth of pubic hair, elevated DHEA levels and hyperinsulinemia, are at high risk for developing the full PCOS phenotype, including ovarian hyperandrogenism and chronic anovulation [4].

Diagnosis

The great variation in the presenting signs and symptoms has lead to many difficulties in the formulation of uniform diagnostic criteria for PCOS. Clinicians and researchers have been using different definitions and uniformity has been conspicuously absent making comparisons of data almost impossible. A meeting in Rotterdam in 2003 has created a consensus proposal [5] and it is recommended that this be used forthwith. Any 2 of the following will make the diagnosis of PCOS:

1. Oligo- or anovulation.
2. Hyperandrogenism – clinical and/or biochemical.
3. Polycystic ovaries.

Other disorders with a similar presentation, congenital adrenal hyperplasia, Cushing's syndrome and androgen secreting tumors, should be excluded.

Investigations

Needless to say, thorough history taking and physical examination are essential. Oligo- or amenorrhea accompanied by symptoms of hyperandrogenism such as hirsutism or persistent acne, virtually make the diagnosis. The typical ultrasound features of the polycystic ovary, 12 or more follicles of 2–8 mm diameter and/or an ovarian volume of $>10\,cm^3$ [5] are best seen using the vaginal route but can be amply viewed transabdominally in adolescents.

The biochemical features of PCOS are very heterogeneous and inconsistent and therefore cannot be relied upon for the diagnosis of the syndrome. They may include increased serum concentrations of testosterone, androstendione and LH and low sex hormone binding globulin (SHBG, <35 nmol/l) as well as evidence of insulin resistance. An estimation of serum testosterone is helpful if an androgen producing tumor is suspected; 17-hydroxy-progesterone concentrations can rule out congenital adrenal hyperplasia to a large extent and Cushing's syndrome, if suspected, can be confirmed in the usual fashion.

While insulin resistance and impaired glucose intolerance are not essential features of the diagnosis, their unveiling may be important at an early stage for the prevention of future health hazards. For obese adolescents or those with a family history of diabetes, screening can be performed relatively easily by employing a fasting glucose:insulin ratio of <7 as a useful index of insulin resistance in adolescents [6]. Regular checks with a 2-hour oral glucose challenge test and fasting lipid profiles should be contemplated as part of the future management of this particular subgroup.

Prevalence

It has been estimated in adults that PCOS occurs in some 5–10% of women in the fertile age group. Data on the prevalence of PCOS in adolescence is very limited but there is no reason to suspect that this is any different to that in adult life as the symptoms are mostly obvious during this early period in life. In the fertile age group, 92% of women presenting with hirsutism had polycystic ovaries diagnosed by ultrasound scanning as had 87% of those presenting with oligomenorrhea and 26% of those with amenorrhea [7].

More than 50% of adolescents who had PCOS have moderate to severe acne [8]. The vast majority of women who have acne have polycystic ovaries as seen from a large study [9] which examined the ultrasound appearance of the ovaries in 82 females referred to a dermatology clinic with acne vulgaris as the presenting symptom. Of these 82 women, 68 (83%) had polycystic ovaries. This staggering figure compares with 19% of women in a control group with no acne who had polycystic ovaries on ultrasound examination. Smaller studies [10] have found a prevalence of ultrasound diagnosed polycystic ovaries in 52–80% of women with persistent, moderate to severe acne. To my mind, these types of study have revolutionized much of the treatment of acne, by informing and emphasizing for dermatologists and gynecologists alike, the role of PCOS in its etiology and applying anti-androgenic therapeutic principles accordingly.

Regarding the prevalence of menstrual disturbances in PCOS, using ultrasonically diagnosed polycystic ovaries as the marker [11] 29.7% had normal cycles, 47% oligomenorrhea, 19.2% amenorrhea, 2.7% polymenorrhea and 1.4% menorrhagia. A similar study that examined the prevalence of menstrual disturbance in women who had both ultrasound features of polycystic ovaries and clinical and/or biochemical evidence of hyperandrogenism [12] found almost identical results in that 73.6% had oligo/amenorrhea and 26.4% had regular menses. Clearly, in adolescents, menstrual disturbance is a very prevalent presenting feature of PCOS and polycystic ovaries are found in the vast majority of adolescents with persistent oligomenorrhea.

Pathophysiology

An overproduction of ovarian androgens is the primary dysfunction in PCOS. Ovarian androgen production is basically dictated by the level of activity of the enzyme cytochrome p450c17α whose actions are mediated by the enzymes 17-hydroxylase and 19.20 lyase. The activity of p450c17α is, in turn, influenced by LH and particularly in PCOS, by the combination of insulin and LH which hyperactivates the enzyme. The amount of free (bioavailable) testosterone in the circulation is regulated by SHBG whose levels are decreased by both high insulin and high androgen concentrations. It is the amount of biologically active free testosterone (normally about 1% of total testosterone) that dictates the severity of the clinical symptoms and even small changes in the concentration of SHBG can make a significant difference. Alternatively, hyperandrogenism may be expressed as a result not of elevated androgen levels but rather of increased sensitivity of the pilosebaceous unit to androgen. This is the probable explanation of the ethnic and genetic differences in the incidence of hirsutism in PCOS which, for example, is much lower in Asian women.

Androgens are known to play a central role in the etiology of acne and hirsutism and increased concentrations of testosterone, androstendione, dehydroepiandrosterone (DHEA) and its sulfate (DHEAS) from ovarian and/or adrenal origin and testosterone and its 5α-reduced metabolite, dihydrotestosterone (DHT), as target-tissue produced androgens have all been implicated.

High androgen concentrations have a deleterious effect on the development, growth and activity of the sebaceous glands and hair follicles. Testosterone is a strong androgen which binds to intracellular androgen receptors in the skin and is converted by 5α-reductase to DHT which has even more potent androgen effects on the hair follicle and sebaceous gland.

Increased sebaceous gland function is of major importance in the etiology of acne. Fueled by overstimulation of the androgen receptors, an excess of sebum is produced. Following this, there are changes in the pattern of follicular keratinization with cornification of the infrainfundibulum of the sebaceous gland. This results in impaired drainage and consequently, the formation of comedones. Abnormal microbial colonization of the pilosebaceous duct by *Proprionibacterium acnes* is the next step down the acne pathway which terminates in inflammation.

Although acne and hirsutism are both androgen driven conditions, both involving the single morphological entity of the pilosebaceous unit and quite often presenting simultaneously, especially in PCOS, they do not always appear concomitantly. It was hypothesized therefore that there may be some dichotomy in the final pathway of endocrine pathogenesis and, indeed it was found that dihydrotestosterone is further reduced to 3α-androstanediol and its glucuroneride only in hirsute patients but not in acne patients [13]. It was concluded that dihydrotestosterone may undergo different metabolic pathways at skin level, supporting the hypothesis that the two clinical entities may be expressions of the different metabolic fate of dihydrotestosterone itself.

The etiology of acne in early adolescence has been associated with increasing serum levels of DHEAS whereas hirsutism has been more directly linked with high concentrations of free testosterone. The two structures comprising the pilosebaceous unit may have different degrees of sensitivity to similar androgenic stimulation [13].

The hormonal profile of women who have acne and ultrasonically demonstrated polycystic ovaries compared with women who have acne but morphologically normal ovaries differs [10]. Those with polycystic ovaries had raised concentrations of androstendione, DHEA, DHEAS, and LH:FSH ratio compared to those with normal ovaries. However, within the group of women with polycystic ovaries, hormonal levels differ. In a large group of women with polycystic ovaries, those with acne alone were much less likely to have the biochemical features of PCOS (e.g. raised LH and testosterone concentrations) compared to those who had hirsutism and other non-dermatological manifestations of PCOS.

The presence and severity of menstrual disturbances have variously been associated with a number of factors. These include obesity, insulin resistance, androgen and LH concentrations and the size of the follicle cohort.

Insulin sensitivity is significantly decreased in women with PCOS with oligomenorrhea compared with women with PCOS but regular cycles and compared with controls with normal ovaries [12]. The combination of insulin insensitivity and polycystic ovaries is thus associated with anovulation and irregular cycles. Menstrual irregularity may be related to the magnitude of insulin sensitivity or insulin secretion [14].

High LH concentrations have also been associated with menstrual irregularity. In a series of 1,741 women with ultrasonically detected polycystic ovaries, those with LH concentrations >10 IU/l had a very significantly increased incidence of cycle disturbance compared with those who had an LH concentration <10 IU/l [11]. In adolescents, hypersecretion of LH is the most common abnormality in those with oligomenorrhea with or without hyperandrogenism.

Treatment

The stigmata of hyperandrogenism can be devastating to a young woman. Hirsutism and acne are blatantly obvious and may have an often disturbing effect on the social life and psychological make up of a teenager. In addition, hyperandrogenism will often upset menstrual rhythm, hinder ovulation and consequently cause infertility. Long-term sequelae of hyperandrogenism, often accompanied by hyperinsulinemia, are now coming to light and failure to relate to the symptoms and signs at an early stage may threaten general health over the age of 40. The management options in adolescent PCOS are numerous, usually symptomatic and, possibly, preventative. Weight loss for the obese and treatment with anti-androgens are well established whereas the use of insulin sensitizers for adolescents with PCOS is still a debatable topic.

Weight Loss and Life Style Changes

Obese adolescents with PCOS have insulin resistance and a consequent hyperinsulinemia. They almost inevitably have the stigmata of hyperandrogenism and irregular menstruation. Insulin stimulates LH and ovarian androgen secretion and decreases SHBG [15]. In addition, high levels of insulin lower insulin-like growth factor binding protein I (IGFBP-I) concentrations, releasing more free IGF-1 which in turn promotes the action of LH. Central obesity and BMI are major determinants of insulin resistance, hyperinsulinemia and hyperandrogenemia.

Just as obesity expresses and exacerbates the signs and symptoms of insulin resistance, then loss of weight can reverse this process by improving ovarian function and the associated hormonal abnormalities. Adolescence is a window for education compared with the difficulties of resetting the life-style of adults. The opportunity to correct eating and life-style habits in these youngsters must be taken as it is excellent strategy in order to achieve short and long term goals such as reduction in hirsutism and acne, return of ovulation and later, conception and almost certainly, a decreased prevalence of cardiovascular disease, hypertension and diabetes mellitus in later life. Curiously, in obese women with PCOS, a loss of 5–10% of body weight is enough to restore reproductive function in 55–100% [16, 17] and greatly improve hirsutism in 40–55% within 6 months of weight reduction [17]. This weight loss can be successfully achieved with a low calorie diet, exercise and a change in lifestyle. Weight loss has the undoubted advantages of being effective and cheap with no side effects.

Insulin Lowering Agents

Metformin is an oral biguanide used for the treatment of diabetes for many years. It is an antihyperglycemic which inhibits hepatic glucose production in hyperglycemic but not euglycemic patients and increases the number of insulin receptors. Insulin concentrations are therefore decreased as a secondary phenomenon with a resulting decrease in androgen and LH concentrations and increase in SHBG. Metformin may also have a direct action on theca cells reducing androgen production. There are now many reports of clinical improvement with metformin in, mostly obese, adult women with PCOS. In doses of 1,500–2,550 mg/day, gastrointestinal side effects have proved troublesome and common in adults but serious side effects have not been reported in an adolescent population [18].

Adolescents with PCOS are inevitably disturbed by the blatant stigmata of acne and hirsutism, and are worried by menstrual irregularity or absence of menstruation but the long-term sequelae of the syndrome are of less immediate concern to them. A debate has now evolved regarding the use of insulin sensitizing agents, notably metformin, in this age group [19, 20]. Theoretically, this treatment, as evidenced in adults, will reduce hyperandrogenism and therefore will improve hirsutism, acne and ovulatory dysfunction in the short to medium term. In the long-term, it would hypothetically help to prevent the onset of type II diabetes, beta cell exhaustion and maybe cardiovascular disease after the age of 40, by eliminating persistent hyperinsulinemia. While traditional treatments with oral contraceptives and anti-androgens correct menstrual irregularity and hyperandrogenemia and consequently acne and hirsutism, they do not positively affect hyperinsulinemia and its consequences.

The question of whether to employ metformin as part of the therapeutic armamentarium in adolescent PCOS is a difficult one based on today's knowledge. There are no large, randomized, controlled trials in adolescents. A handful of studies, short-term and with small numbers, have shown a distinct improvement in obese and non-obese adolescents with PCOS in restoring menstrual regularity and improving androgen concentrations. Glueck et al. [21] gave metformin for a mean of 10 months to 11 oligo- or amenorrheic adolescents with PCOS. Ten responded by resuming regular, ovulatory cycles. Although this sounds encouraging, the results are confounded by a concomitant diet-induced weight reduction. Ibanez et al. [22] gave metformin for 6 months to

18 non-obese girls with anovulatory, hyperinsulinemic hyperandrogenism with success in that 14 started ovulating regularly and no serious side effects were noted. A recent study by the same team [23] examined the effects of a low-dose combination of flutamide and metformin on 30 teenagers who had hyperinsulinemic hyperandrogenism. Hirsutism, serum androgens, insulin sensitivity, lipid profile, abdominal fat and ovulation rate all showed marked improvement on this treatment.

Several questions still remain unanswered. Is metformin effective in preventing the long-term sequelae of the syndrome? Will it prove as completely safe as present data suggest? What will be the effect of committing a teenager to maybe 20 years of medication? Well-controlled, randomized, long-term trials are needed to answer these questions. A further question relates to the fact that a correct diet and life style have already proven value in the prevention of diabetes, hypertension and cardio-vascular disease in adults. Can this kind of education be impressed upon adolescent girls with PCOS and continued into the reproductive years? If so, there is much to be gained.

Anti-Androgens

As acne and hirsutism associated with PCOS undoubtedly arise from over stimulation of the pilosebaceous unit by androgens, then anti-androgens are the most effective long-term treatment option. Although anti-androgens are today the cornerstone of the treatment, more traditional dermatological treatment is still being used, either alone or combined with anti-androgen therapy. These include antibiotics, administered either topically or systemically, usually tetracyclines in combination with topical benzoyl peroxide 5% or tretinoin, widely prescribed by dermatologists.

A number of anti-androgen medications that block the synthesis or action of androgens: cyproterone acetate (CPA), spironolactone, flutamide or finasteride are employed today.

Excluding North America, a combination of CPA (an orally active progestogen) and ethinyl estradiol (EE) is probably the most widely used anti-androgen. CPA has an anti-androgen action at several sites: (1) In combination with EE, suppression of LH release by the anterior pituitary. (2) Competition for the androgen receptor which it blocks. (3) As a progestogen in suppressing the action of 5α-reductase. (4) With EE, increases SHBG concentrations. The combination of CPA (2 mg/day) and EE (35 μg/day) given cyclically has proved very effective in the treatment of hirsutism and acne as well as serving as an excellent contraceptive. A reduction of more than 50% in the hirsutism score has been demonstrated after 9 months of treatment and acne has been successfully treated in almost 100% of cases using this minimal dose [24]. The addition of CPA in a dose of 10–100 mg/day on the first 10 days of the combined medication has proved effective for more severe cases. Success rates in reversing or severely diminishing symptoms and maintaining improvement with minimal side effects are high but patients need to be informed that this treatment is not 'instant' and that at least 4–9 months are needed to see an improvement in hirsutism and 3–5 months for acne. Acne will be cleared in 60% of patients in 6 months and after 12 months, 95% should be completely free. Side effects of CPA in combination with ethinyl estradiol are similar to those of oral contraceptives, are usually mild and transient and include mastodinia, increased appetite and headaches. No adverse effects on insulin metabolism or lipid levels by CPA were recorded in a 1-year trial [25].

Other anti-androgens, spironolactone, flutamide and finesteride are also being employed, mainly in North America where CPA is unavailable. However, they are not well established therapeutic options for PCOS and for adolescent PCOS in particular.

However effective these anti-androgen medicines may be, they ameliorate symptoms while they are being taken but fail to 'cure' the cause. After the withdrawal of treatment with spironolactone, flutamide or CPA, hirsutism relapses to 60–80% of the original score, regardless of which anti-androgen therapy is used [26]. However, the longer the duration of treatment with CPA/EE, the less chance of relapse within a given time. Using long term treatment with CPA (25–50 mg/day) and EE (0.01–0.02 mg/day) in a reverse sequential regimen, hirsutism was absent for 6 months following cessation of treatment in all patients [27]. After 12 months without treatment, 28% had worsened and after 24 months, 44% were still showing an improvement on the original hirsutism score.

The full compliance of the adolescent on anti-androgen treatment is very much dependent on the accuracy and fullness of information given to her by the physician. First and foremost, the information that a good clinical response to treatment takes time must be explained. Secondly, the need for long-term maintenance treatment of 3–4 years, even when obvious clinical improvement has been achieved. Thirdly, the possibility of relapse some time after treatment is terminated.

The aim of treatment for the menstrual disturbances associated with PCOS is to provide a regular menstrual cycle. This can be achieved using measures which will also relieve symptoms associated with hyperandrogenism, particularly hirsutism and acne, will prevent endometrial hyperplasia and may help prevent long-term health consequences.

As with the treatment of all other symptoms associated with PCOS in obese patients, weight loss should be the first line of treatment. This alone has an excellent chance of restoring normal menstrual regularity in patients who succeed in losing >5% of their body weight [16]. This improvement is associated with a reduction in circulating insulin and androgen levels which can also be achieved using insulin sensitizing drugs. Metformin improves cyclicity in about 50% of patients with oligo/amenorrhea (see above). In a compilation of data from controlled trials, Harborne et al. [28] found that women on metformin had 41 cycles per 100 patient months compared with 21 cycles per patient months in those receiving placebo. They concluded that these improvements were variable and modest. It seems therefore that insulin sensitizers cannot yet be recommended as treatment for adolescent PCOS when menstrual irregularity is the sole complaint.

For symptoms of hyperandrogenism associated with their menstrual irregularity, the cyclical administration of CPA/EE would seem to be the optimal treatment. This has been described at length above. As untreated PCOS may be regarded as a progressive syndrome, at least up to the age of 40, it is reasonable to assume that treatment with this combination of EE and CPA, which markedly reduces androgen concentrations and their untoward effects, will put the syndrome 'on hold' so improving the prospects of success of fertility treatment when it is discontinued. All other cyclically administered contraceptive pills will of course regularize the cycle.

Conclusions

Persistent oligomenorrhea is a common symptom of PCOS in adolescence and PCOS also underlies many a case of moderate to severe acne and hirsutism. Awareness of the early symptoms of PCOS is essential for diagnosis and correct symptomatic management. The combination of cyproterone acetate and ethinyl estradiol is very effective for the treatment of acne, hirsutism and cycle disturbances. Treatment with insulin sensitizers for the adolescent is a possibility but not yet scientifically established; for the obese adolescent, loss of weight is equally as effective.

References

1 Van Hooff MHA, Voorhoorst FJ, Kaptein MBH, Hirasing RA, Koppenaal C, Schoemaker J: Endocrine features of polycystic ovary syndrome in a random population sample 14- to 16-year-old adolescents. Hum Reprod 1999;14:2223–2229.

2 Siegberg R, Nilsson CG, Stenman UH, Widhold O: Endocrinologic features of oligomenorrheic adolescent girls. Fertil Steril 1986;46:852–857.

3 Apter D, Vihko R: Endocrine determinants of fertility: Serum androgen concentrations during follow-up of adolescents into the third decade of life. J Clin Endocrinol Metab 1990;71:970–974.

4 Legro RS: Detection of insulin resistance and its treatment in adolescents with polycystic ovary syndrome. J Pediatr Endocrinol Metab 2002;15(suppl 5):1367–1378.

5 The Rotterdam ESHRE/ASRM-Sponsored PCOS Consensus Workshop Group: Revised 2003 consensus on diagnostic criteria and long-term health risks related to polycystic ovary syndrome (PCOS). Hum Reprod 2004;9:41–47.
6 Kent SC, Legro RS: Polycystic ovary syndrome in adolescents. Adolesc Med 2002;13:73–88.
7 Adams J, Polson DW, Franks S: Prevalence of polycystic ovaries in women with anovulation and idiopathic hirsutism. Br Med J 1986;293:355–359.
8 Dramusic V, Rajan U, Wong YC, Chan P, Ratnam SIS, Wong YC: Adolescent polycystic ovary syndrome. Ann NY Acad Sci 1997;816:194–208.
9 Bunker CB, Newton J, Kilborn J, Patel A, Conway GS, Jacobs HS, Greaves MW, Dowd PM: Most women with acne have polycystic ovaries. Br J Dermatol 1989;121:675–680.
10 Betti R, Bencini PL, Lodi A, Urbani CE, Chiarelli G, Crosti C: Incidence of polycystic ovaries in patients with late onset or persistent acne: Hormonal reports. Dermatologica 1990;181:109–111.
11 Balen AH, Conway GS, Kaltsas G, Techatrasak K, Manning PJ, West C, Jacobs HS: Polycystic ovary syndrome: The spectrum of the disorder in 1741 patients. Hum Reprod 1995;10:2705–2712.
12 Robinson S, Kiddy D, Gelding SV, Willis D, Nithanthian R, Bush A, Johnston DG, Franks S: The relationship of insulin insensitivity to menstrual pattern in women with hyperandrogenism and polycystic ovaries. Clin Endocrinol 1993;39:351–355.
13 Toscano V, Balducci R, Bianchi P, Guglielmi R, Mangiantini A, Rossi FG, Colonna LM, Sciarra F: Two different pathogenic mechanisms may play a role in acne and in hirsutism. Clin Endocrinol (Oxf) 1993;39:551–556.
14 Legro RS, Bentley-Lewis R, Driscoll D, Wang SC, Dunaif A: Insulin resistance in the sisters of women with polycystic ovary syndrome: Association with hyperandrogenemia rather than menstrual irregularity. J Clin Endocrinol Metab 2002;87:2128–2133.
15 Poretsky L, Cataldo NA, Rosenwaks Z, Giudice LC: The insulin related ovarian regulatory system in health and disease. Endocr Rev 1999;20:535–582.
16 Kiddy DS, Hamilton-Fairley D, Bush A, Short F, Anyaoku V, Reed MJ, Franks S: Improvement in endocrine and ovarian function during dietary treatment of obese women with polycystic ovary syndrome. Clin Endocrinol 1992;36:105–111.
17 Pasquali R, Antenucci D, Casmirri F, Venturoli S, Paradisi R, Fabbri R, Balestra V, Melchionda N, Barbara L: Clinical and hormonal characteristics of obese amenorrheic hyperandrogenic women before and after weight loss. J Clin Endocrinol Metab 1989;68:173–179.
18 Legro RS: Polycystic ovary syndrome: Current and future treatment paradigms. Am J Obstet Gynecol 1998;1795:S101.
19 Jamieson MA: The use of metformin in adolescents with polycystic ovary syndrome. J Pediatr Adolesc Gynecol 2002;15:109–114.
20 Homburg R, Lambalk CB: Polycystic ovary syndrome in adolescence: A therapeutic conundrum. Hum Reprod 2004;19:1039–1042.
21 Glueck CJ, Wang P, Fontaine R, Tracy T, Sieve-Smith L: Metformin to restore normal menses in oligo-amenorrheic teenage girls with polycystic ovary syndrome. J Adolesc Health 2001;29:160–169.
22 Ibanez L, Valls C, Ferrer A, Marcos MV, Rodriguez-Hiero F, de Zegher F: Sensitization to insulin induces ovulation in nonobese adolescents with anovulatory hyperandrogenism. J Clin Endocrinol Metab 2001;86:3595–3598.
23 Ibanez L, Ong K, Ferrer A, Amin R, Dunger D, de Zegher F: Low dose flutamide-metformin therapy reverses insulin resistance and reduces fat mass in nonobese adolescents with ovarian hyperandrogenism. J Clin Endocrinol Metab 2003;88:2600–2606.
24 Van Waygen RG, van den Ende A: Experience in the long term treatment of hisutism and/or acne with cyproterone acetate-containing preparations. Efficacy, metabolic and endocrine effects. Exp Clin Endocrinol Diab 1995;103:241–251.
25 Harborne L, Fleming R, Lyall H, Sattar N, Norman J: Metformin or antiandrogen in the treatment of hirsutism in polycystic ovary syndrome. J Clin Endocrinol Metab 2003;88:4116–4123.
26 Yucelten D, Erenus M, Gurbuz O, Durmusoglu F: Recurrence rate of hirsutism after 3 different anti-androgen therapies. J Am Acad Dermatol 1999;41:64–68.

27 Flagmini C, Venturoli S, Fabbri R: Long term management of hirsute patients with cyproterone acetate; in Spona J, Aydinlik S (eds): Hirsutism and Endocrine Dermatological Problems. Carnforth, Parthenon Press, 1988, pp 29–37.
28 Harborne L, Fleming R, Lyall H, Norman J, Sattar N: Descriptive review of the evidence for the use of metformin in polycystic ovary syndrome. Lancet 2003;361:1894–1900.

Prof. Roy Homburg
Division of Reproductive Medicine, Department of Obstetrics and Gynaecology
De Boelelaan 1117, Postbus 7057, NL–1007 MB Amsterdam (The Netherlands)
Tel. +31 0 20 444 0070, Fax +31 0 20 444 0045, E-Mail r.homburg@vumc.nl

Delemarre-van de Waal HA (ed): Abnormalities in Puberty. Scientific and Clinical Advances.
Endocr Dev. Basel, Karger, 2005, vol 8, pp 150–165

Reversing Sex Steroid Deficiency and Optimizing Skeletal Development in the Adolescent with Gonadal Failure

Dirk Vanderschueren[a], *Liesbeth Vandenput*[a], *Steven Boonen*[a,b]

[a]Laboratory for Experimental Medicine and Endocrinology, and
[b]Leuven University Centre for Metabolic Bone Diseases and Division of Geriatric Medicine, Katholieke Universiteit Leuven, Leuven, Belgium

Abstract

During puberty, the acquisition of skeletal mass and areal bone mineral density (BMD) mainly reflects an increase in bone size (length and perimeters) and not true volumetric BMD. Sexual dimorphism in bone mass and areal BMD is also explained by differences in bone size (longer and wider bones in males) and not by differences in volumetric BMD. Androgens stimulate skeletal growth by activation of the androgen receptor, whereas estrogens (following aromatization of androgens and stimulation of estrogen receptors) have a biphasic effect on skeletal growth during puberty. Recent evidence from clinical cases has shown that many of the growth-promoting effects of the sex steroids are mediated through estrogens rather than androgens. In addition, skeletal maturation and epiphyseal fusion are also estrogen-dependent in both sexes. Nevertheless, independent actions of androgens in these processes also occur. Both sex steroids maintain volumetric BMD during puberty. Androgens interact with the growth hormone (GH)–insulin-like growth factor-I (IGF-I) axis neonatally, resulting in a sexual dimorphic GH pattern during puberty, whereas estrogens stimulate GH and hereby IGF-I in both sexes. Hypogonadism in adolescents impairs not only bone size but also maintenance of volumetric BMD, hereby severely reducing peak areal BMD. Delayed puberty in boys and Turner's syndrome in women impair both bone length and size, reducing areal BMD. Whether volumetric BMD is also reduced and whether fracture risk is increased in these conditions remains controversial. Replacing sex steroids according to a biphasic pattern (starting at low doses and ending at high-normal doses) seems the safest approach to reach targeted height and to optimize bone development.

Puberty has a fundamental role in the development of the skeleton. Indeed, skeletal mass approximately doubles between the onset of puberty and young adulthood. This accelerated skeletal growth and modeling is needed because of increased mechanical demands imposed upon the skeleton. The pubertal increase in growth velocity and accumulation of bone mass are regulated by the interactions between sex steroids, growth hormone (GH), and insulin-like growth factor-I (IGF-I), along with nutritional and environmental factors [1, 2]. The accrual of bone mass during puberty is a major determinant of peak bone mass, and, therefore, of the risk of osteoporotic fractures occurring later in life. Puberty thus represents a vulnerable period during which a deficiency or even a delay of sex steroid action may irreversibly impact on bone mass and structure. During puberty, both androgens and estrogens have anabolic effects on the skeleton. Sex steroids predominantly stimulate bone formation through direct activation of sex steroid receptors [androgen receptor (AR), estrogen receptor-α (ERα), ERβ] in different bone cells and compartments. In addition, they may also exert their effects indirectly through interaction with the GH-IGF-I axis as well as by mechanical stimulation following muscle growth. In this chapter, we will review the role of sex steroids in the skeletal changes during puberty.

Bone Development during Puberty

During childhood and adolescence, bone mass and bone mineral density (BMD) increase in boys and girls, with a maximal accumulation of BMD at the lumbar spine and femoral neck in the final stages of puberty (fig. 1a) [3]. The enhancement of BMD is mainly caused by the increase in bone size, leading to a proportional increase in bone mineral. During puberty, sex differences in bone width are established. This sexual dimorphism of the skeleton is characterized by a larger bone size in males, with both a larger diameter and greater cortical thickness. This is the result of increased periosteal bone formation in men, with less periosteal apposition in women. At the endocortical site, men experience greater expansion during puberty, whereas in females endocortical contraction occurs, narrowing the marrow cavity (fig. 2) [4]. Growth velocity is different during childhood and adolescence in the different regions of the skeleton. Before puberty, appendicular growth remains more rapid than axial growth. At puberty, sex steroid production slows long bone growth by epiphyseal fusion and accelerates axial growth [5]. This differing pattern of growth between axial and appendicular sites will cause site-specific deficits in case of illness. Exposure to illness during the prepubertal period will affect the dimensions of the appendicular skeleton. In contrast, illness during pubertal years, e.g. delayed or deficient sex steroid production, will enhance epiphyseal growth resulting in longer leg length whereas the failure of the axial growth spurt produces a short trunk. This

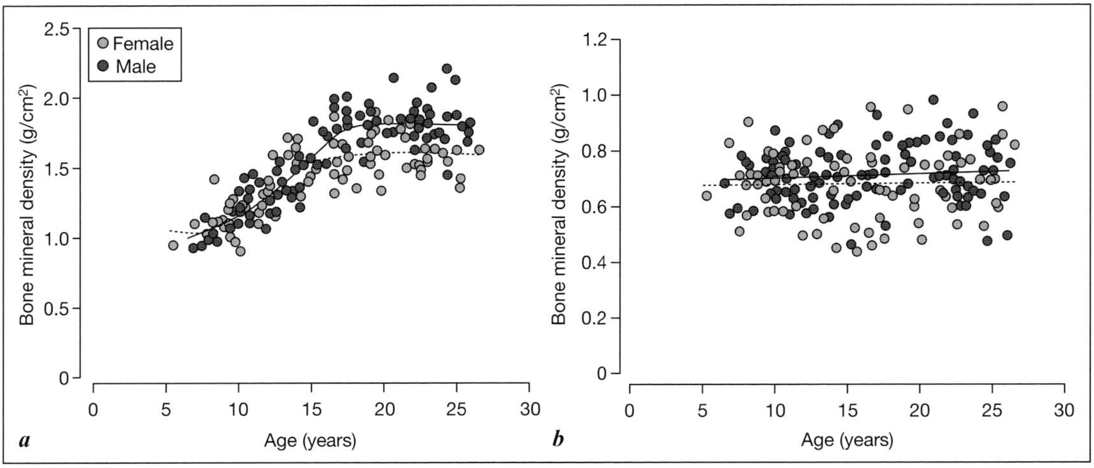

Fig. 1. Femoral shaft areal (***a***) and volumetric (***b***) bone mineral density in men and women. Reproduced with permission from Lu et al. [3]. ©The Endocrine Society.

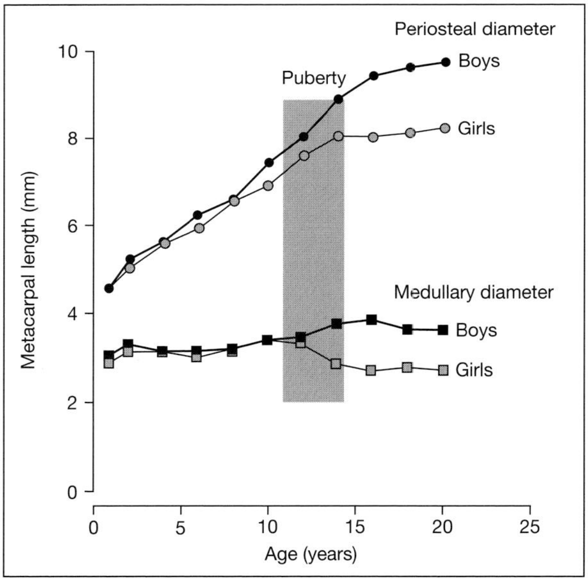

Fig. 2. Effects of puberty on bone development in boys and girls. Reproduced with permission from Seeman [4]. ©Elsevier.

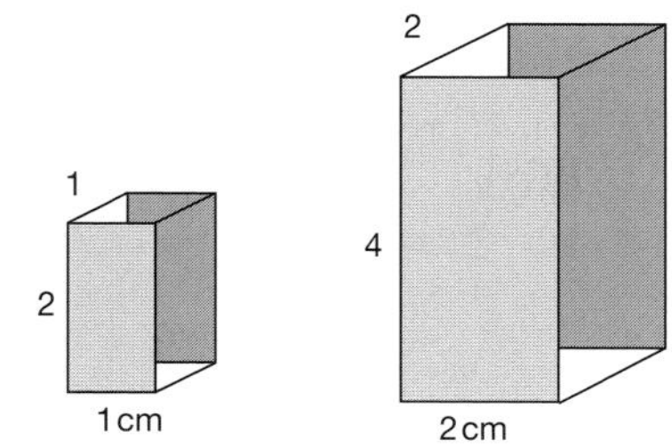

	1 cm	2 cm
Volumetric bone density (g/cm^3)	1.0	1.0
Volume (cm^3)	2.0	16.0
Areal BMC (g)	2.0	16.0
Projected area (cm^2)	2.0	8.0
Areal BMD (mg/cm^2)	1.0	2.0

Fig. 3. Effect of object size on commonly measured bone mineral parameters. Using densitometry techniques based on a 2-dimensional projection of a 3-dimensional structure, the region of interest or projected area is equal to the front face of the sample. The bone mineral content (BMC) is the total amount of bone mineral in the sample. The areal density is calculated as BMC over a projected area. The areal BMD of the larger sample is twice that of the smaller sample. Volumetric BMD, however, is similar in both samples. Reproduced with permission from Carter et al. [7]. ©The American Society for Bone and Mineral Research.

so-called eunuchoid phenotype is well documented in Klinefelter's syndrome (KS) and aromatase deficiency (see below). The timing of pubertal growth is also sex-specific. Since boys enter puberty at a later age, and thus have a longer prepubertal (appendicular) growth period and longer pubertal growth spurt, they achieve greater height and have longer bones than girls [6]. As a result, at the end of puberty males have longer and wider bones compared to females. Areal BMD at the end of puberty, expressed as the bone mineral content over the projected area and measured by dual-energy X-ray absorptiometry (DXA), is greater in men compared to women (fig. 1a). This is due to the fact that men have a larger bone size, not a denser bone. Volumetric bone density, expressed as the bone mineral content over the bone volume, is similar in both sexes in long bones and independent of age (fig. 1b). Volumetric trabecular BMD of the spine remains independent of age until puberty, when it increases to a similar degree in both boys and girls. Bone density assessments by methods which rely on two-dimensional projection of a three-dimensional structure are largely influenced by the size of the region and should therefore be interpreted with caution (fig. 3) [7]. These techniques may overestimate the bone mineral deficit during growth in patients with altered growth patterns. Relevant clinical examples of such discrepancies between volumetric and areal bone density are delayed puberty in boys and Turner's syndrome (TS) in girls (see further).

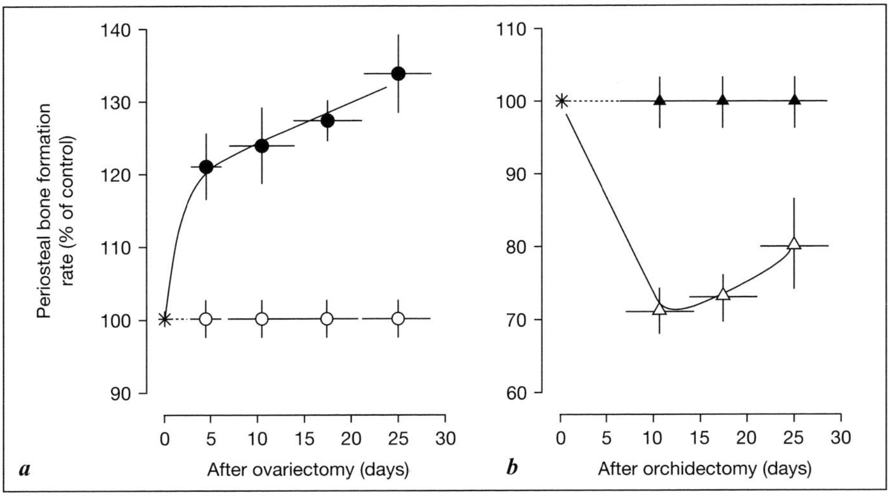

Fig. 4. ***a*** The effect of ovariectomy on periosteal bone formation rate. The mean ± SE (vertical bar) and tetracycline labeling period (horizontal line) for intact controls (○) and ovariectomized (●) rats are shown as a function of time after ovariectomy. $p < 0.01$ for all time points compared to intact controls. ***b*** The effect of orchidectomy on periosteal bone formation rate. The mean ± SE and tetracycline labeling period for intact controls (▲) and orchidectomized rats (△) are shown as a function of time after orchidectomy. $p < 0.01$ for all orch time points compared to the same labeling period in intact controls. Reproduced with permission from Turner et al. [10].

Effects of Sex Steroids on Bone Mass during Puberty

During pubertal development, rising concentrations of androgens and estrogens enhance longitudinal growth in boys and girls, respectively, either directly or indirectly by stimulating GH secretion. At the end of puberty, higher concentrations of estrogens induce growth plate closure in both sexes [8]. In boys, cortical width increases by periosteal apposition, which is mediated by androgens, whereas estrogens inhibit periosteal bone formation, resulting in a smaller bone in girls. The endocortical apposition in females, narrowing the marrow cavity, is regulated by estrogens and probably dependent on the GH-IGF-I axis [9]. Accordingly, studies in orchidectomized and ovariectomized rodent models have shown that androgens stimulate periosteal bone formation whereas estrogens inhibit periosteal expansion (fig. 4) [10].

Role of Aromatization of Androgens in Estrogens

Androgens have the unique feature that they can be converted into estrogens, even within bone (fig. 5). Recently, the pivotal role of estrogens in male skeletal

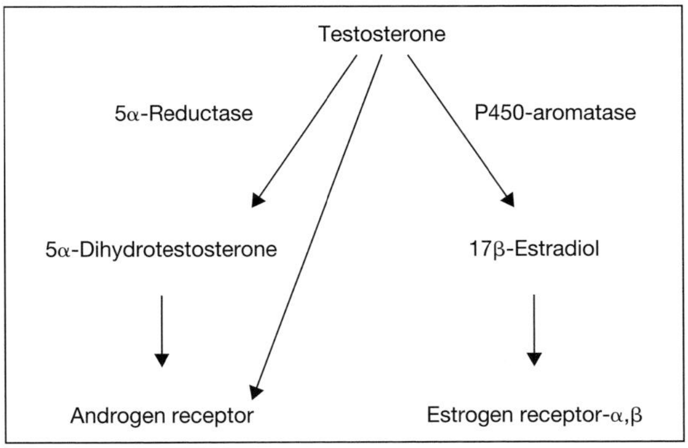

Fig. 5. Metabolism of testosterone. Testosterone may activate the androgen receptor either directly or indirectly following transformation by the 5α-reductase enzyme into the non-aromatizable androgen dihydrotestosterone. Alternatively, it can be converted into 17β-estradiol via aromatization and activate one or both estrogen receptors.

development and maintenance has received much attention [for extensive review see 11]. Indeed, men suffering from estrogen deficiency (due to a mutation in the aromatase gene) or resistance (secondary to a mutation in the ERα gene) have delayed skeletal maturation and impaired bone mass, resulting in low areal bone density. In addition, these patients do not experience a pubertal growth spurt but continue to grow into adulthood. Treatment of aromatase deficient men with estrogens increases skeletal maturation. This indicates that androgens alone are not sufficient for epiphyseal maturation and skeletal mineralization in boys and that estrogens appear crucial for pubertal growth, acquisition of peak bone mass and epiphyseal fusion not only in girls but also in boys [12].

A dual mode of action of androgens on bone via both the ER and AR pathways is now well established [13]. During male hypogonadism, the degree of estrogen deficiency may vary according to the capacity to aromatize androgens. Patients with very low androgens also have limited capacity for aromatization. Male hypogonadism should therefore be regarded as a combination of varying degrees of androgen and estrogen deficiency, which may impact differently on bone.

Effects of Androgens Mediated Directly via the Androgen Receptor

The role of aromatization of androgens into estrogens in skeletal mineralization and epiphyseal fusion in boys has been well established. Therefore, the question arises to what extent androgens affect skeletal development directly via the AR. Clear evidence for the contribution of androgens to male skeletal development and maintenance comes from men affected by the complete androgen insensitivity syndrome (cAIS). Low areal bone density at the hip and spine is a frequent finding in these phenotypically female cAIS patients [14–17]. When correcting these DXA measurements for tall stature, the skeletal deficits are even more severe [18]. These findings suggest that androgens may directly stimulate bone density via the AR, not only indirectly after aromatization into estrogens. However, bone density values in androgen-resistant patients may be confounded by surgical castration and (inadequate) hormone replacement therapy [18]. In addition, estrogens increase areal bone density at the spine and hip in most patients with cAIS [16, 17], although these measurements have not always been adjusted for their tall stature. Also, cAIS patients on long-term estrogen replacement therapy still have reduced areal BMD compared to controls, indicating that both androgens and estrogens contribute to peak bone mass. Finally, androgen resistance in humans is not associated with impaired longitudinal growth or an abnormal pubertal growth spurt, providing further evidence for the pivotal role of estrogens in longitudinal bone growth and epiphyseal closure in men [8]. The lack of eunuchoid skeletal development in these patients also supports this view. Whether androgen resistance in men affects periosteal bone formation – as would be expected from animal research – is not known.

Interaction of Sex Steroids with the GH-IGF-I Axis

Prepubertally, GH is essential to longitudinal growth. During puberty, androgens and estrogens increase the spontaneous secretion of GH, initializing the pubertal growth spurt. More importantly, the dynamic interaction between increasing levels of GH and sex steroids determines the acquisition of peak bone mass and skeletal maturation [1]. In general, IGF-I levels are stimulated by sex steroids due to an increased GH secretion. However, especially for estrogens, direct effects on the hepatic IGF-I secretion which are not mediated by GH are also important. Estrogens modulate longitudinal growth in a biphasic manner: low doses of estrogen stimulate IGF-I production, but higher doses inhibit IGF-I production at the hepatic level. Androgens indirectly stimulate IGF-I following aromatization into estrogens at the pituitary [19]. Studies in male rats have confirmed that aromatase inhibitors lower serum levels of IGF-I [20], whereas antiestrogens which do not penetrate the blood-brain barrier do not affect serum IGF-I [21]. Interestingly, non-aromatizable androgens such as dihydrotestosterone and oxandrolone may initiate pubertal growth in boys with delayed puberty without a concomitant increase in serum GH or IGF-I [22]. Taken together, these findings support the view that not only local but also central action of sex steroids on the GH-IGF-I axis may be important for the regulation of skeletal dimensions and bone (re)modeling.

Role of Estrogens and Androgens in Women

As mentioned before, puberty and the associated growth spurt start earlier in girls. This increase is related to an earlier rise of estrogen levels in prepubertal girls compared to prepubertal boys [23]. Pubertal growth spurt and skeletal mineralization precede normal breast development in girls, suggesting that increased growth occurs at even lower estrogen levels than those necessary for the development of secondary sexual characteristics. These very low but biologically active estrogen concentrations can only be measured by an ultrasensitive bioassay and not by conventional immunoassays. It is also clear that the rise of these low but biologically active estrogen levels occurs later in boys, as does their corresponding increase of growth and skeletal development [23]. Most, if not all, of the growth-stimulatory action of these low estrogen levels is mediated by stimulation of GH and IGF-I in girls as well as boys. The GH pattern in girls, however, differs from the one in boys and is characterized by a higher basal secretion with less and lower peaks. After menarche, estrogen levels rise and continued exposure leads to epiphyseal fusion. The exact molecular and cellular mechanism of this process remains to be clarified.

The role of androgens in female skeletal development is not well established. In women, serum androgen concentrations vary considerably: although testosterone concentrations are lower than in men, serum concentrations of other 'weaker' androgens like androstenedione and dehydroepiandrosterone-sulfate are similar [24]. Androgens may therefore stimulate skeletal development during puberty in women and contribute to clinically relevant differences in bone density. Most data in support of such a bone-stimulatory action are based on a number of studies in women suffering from the polycystic ovary syndrome (PCOS) [25 and references therein]. Studies in the PCOS model have provided evidence that hirsute women have higher peak bone density than age-matched controls, even after correction for body mass index [26, 27]. It is important to note that this increase in bone density has been confirmed by cancellous peripheral quantitative computed tomography (pQCT) and, thus, reflects real changes in bone tissue composition, rather than changes in bone size. Still, it remains unclear to what extent adrenal androgens have direct AR-mediated skeletal effects or mainly represent a source for aromatization into estrogens in both sexes.

Effects of Delayed Puberty on Bone in Men

During puberty, delay of androgen production adversely affects skeletal growth, as evidenced by reduced peak bone mass and decreased spinal and femoral areal BMD in patients with constitutional delay of puberty [28–31].

Again, bone density assessments based on projectional methods should be interpreted with caution. These methods may overestimate the bone mineral deficit during growth because of the associated failure to expand bone during delayed puberty. In this regard, measurements of density using (p)QCT are more appropriate. In fact, volumetric BMD in adult men with a history of late puberty tended to be normal in one [32], but not all studies [33], suggesting that the impairment of bone size may be more important in these men than changes in bone tissue composition. Body proportions may also be modified, with long leg length compared to trunk length.

Effects of Gonadal Failure on Skeletal Growth in Men

In young hypogonadal men, skeletal growth is impaired and, therefore, areal BMD will be even more affected than during adult hypogonadism. Isolated hypogonadotropic hypogonadism (IHH) represents the most complete and early form of male hypogonadism. In contrast to most other types of hypogonadotropic hypogonadism, men with IHH have isolated sex steroid deficiency without other metabolic abnormalities, making IHH a good model to examine the effects of sex steroids and sex steroid deficiencies in men. Compared to age-matched controls, patients with IHH have lower bone density at the spine and radius, not only before but also after growth plate closure [34]. Interestingly, both areal and volumetric bone densities are reduced. This suggests that bone size and composition may both be impaired in the context of IHH. In these patients, assessing bone turnover has produced inconsistent results, demonstrating histomorphometric evidence for low-turnover osteoporosis in some patients [35] but increased levels of markers of bone formation and resorption in others [36].

Lower bone density (at radius and spine) is well documented in hyperprolactinemic hypogonadal men as well [37]. Moreover, reversal of the hypogonadism will significantly increase cortical bone density, irrespective of the serum levels of prolactin, suggesting that it is the T deficiency and not prolactin excess which impairs skeletal homeostasis in these patients [38].

Finally, KS is the most frequent form of hypergonadotropic hypogonadism in men. According to most studies – with one exception [39] – bone density (areal BMD as well as calculated volumetric BMD) is decreased in KS [40–44]. Low bone density has even been reported in patients who have already been receiving long-term T replacement [43, 44], questioning the role of androgen deficiency as the cause of the bone deficit (as well as the role of androgen replacement to maintain bone density in this patient group) and suggesting other, disease-specific effects on bone which may be independent of the associated hypogonadism. Varying degrees of hypogonadism have been observed in patients with KS and only those with severe hypogonadism may experience bone loss [39, 42]. However, because of the small numbers of subjects and the lack of appropriate control groups in most studies dealing with KS, controversy is likely to persist until large prospective and controlled studies document the skeletal impact of different degrees of hypogonadism (and their response to T replacement).

Effects of Gonadal Failure on Skeletal Growth in Women

TS is caused by partial or total absence of a second X chromosome and is characterized by ovarian failure, short stature, and multiple skeletal abnormalities [45]. The two latter features have been attributed to haploinsufficiency for SHOX, a pseudoautosomal homeobox gene involved in skeletal development [46].

Early densitometric studies in TS patients have indicated that bone mass is decreased at both cortical (radius) and trabecular (spine) sites [47, 48]. These studies did not account for the variables (height, bone age, body size) that may impact on bone density measurements. Of these factors, correcting for height is particularly important in TS patients. The observed areal BMD reduction is thus likely the result of their impaired growth and hereby reduced bone size. After adjusting for height, bone mass was indeed adequate for bone size, at least at trabecular sites [49–53]. Several studies have recently shown a selective reduction in volumetric BMD at sites with predominantly cortical bone [54–56]. In addition, Bechtold et al. [51], using pQCT, reported decreased cortical bone mass and thickness due to failure of endocortical apposition during puberty in young patients with TS. The reduced amount of cortical bone resulted in a decreased bone strength, which may explain the higher fracture incidence observed in TS patients [49, 57, 58]. In contrast, Bakalov et al. [55] recently reported that the prevalence of osteoporosis and bone fractures is not increased in women with TS who received adequate estrogen therapy.

Management of Gonadal Failure

Hypogonadal boys are treated with sex steroids in order to induce a normal pubertal growth spurt and secondary sex characteristics. Although the skeleton of prepubertal boys already responds to T [59], the benefits of T replacement have been most extensively documented in adult hypogonadal men. The interest of the scientific community in the potential benefits of androgen administration currently extends not only to adult male hypogonadism but also to young men with gonadal failure.

As mentioned earlier, the skeletal effects of gonadal failure during puberty (deficient peak bone mass acquisition and loss of volumetric BMD) will be much more severe than during gonadal failure after peak bone mass acquisition (mainly loss of volumetric BMD). Indeed, peak bone mass acquisition (25% of total bone calcium) occurs shortly after peak growth velocity whereas about 50% of total calcium is accumulated during entire puberty. Unfortunately, the diagnosis of hypogonadism (especially in those with partial hypogonadism) and initiation of treatment is often delayed. Therefore, androgen treatment will inhibit further loss and some gain of volumetric BMD may be expected, but it is unlikely that the expected peak bone mass and bone size will be obtained. Finkelstein et al. [35] have shown that the effect of testosterone treatment on BMD is related to the initial degree of bone maturation. In boys with open epiphyses at the start of the study, both cortical and trabecular BMD increased. Androgen replacement in boys with closed epiphyses only increased cortical BMD and the increase was smaller than in the former group. Neither group, however, attained normalization of BMD after treatment. Although no studies have compared bone mineral acquisition in those receiving early versus late sex steroid replacement, we would currently advise to start sex steroid replacement as soon as possible in order to optimize bone development, even when the differential diagnosis between delayed puberty and hypogonadism is unclear.

Most studies on TS have focused on height optimization. Treatment of TS patients with GH, given alone or in combination with oxandrolone, improves final height [60, 61]. It is tempting to speculate that such treatment not only optimizes height but also bone width and areal bone density. As mentioned earlier, areal BMD, corrected for height, seems normal in TS patients.

If spontaneous puberty seems unlikely in TS, puberty is induced with estrogen replacement therapy at an appropriate bone age, taking into account growth optimization [45]. Trabecular BMD values of women with TS given appropriate estrogen replacement therapy differ little from healthy matched controls [50, 53], suggesting that such replacement maintains volumetric BMD in TS. High-dose subcutaneous E2 implants may even increase trabecular bone volume and wall thickness in young women with TS [62]. However, it is unclear whether such an increase of volumetric BMD is beneficial. A selective reduction in cortical volumetric BMD has recently been reported in TS patients, but this may be related to the chromosomal abnormality per se and not to the treatment they received [54, 56].

Whether postponing estrogen replacement therapy in TS patients (to optimize height) is also optimal for peak bone mass acquisition and skeletal maturation remains to be clarified.

Management of Delayed Puberty

Constitutional delay of growth and puberty represents another potential indication for T therapy [63]. Studies in a small number of adolescents with delayed puberty suggest that monthly injections of low T may increase bone density [29, 64]. However, the ultimate impact of this treatment on adult bone density has not been documented. It is also not clear to what extent such increase in bone density is due to an increase in bone size. According to Bertelloni et al. [32], no differences in areal and volumetric BMD of the spine were found in boys with delayed puberty, either untreated or treated with T.

The nonaromatizable androgen oxandrolone has been reported to increase height gain and bone maturation to the same extent as T in boys with delayed puberty [65, 66]. In boys treated with oxandrolone, the predicted adult height is significantly increased [66]. To date, no data are available on its effect on bone density in these patients, except one study in a small number of patients indicating that neither T nor oxandrolone increases areal or volumetric BMD [32].

Recently, Wickman et al. [67] demonstrated that combined treatment of testosterone and an aromatase inhibitor appears to increase the predicted final height more than testosterone alone by delaying bone maturation and epiphyseal fusion. This type of treatment did not seem to impair peak bone mass acquisition [64], but the number of observations and the duration of the study were limited. In growing male rats, however, aromatase inhibitors impair peak bone mass acquisition and volumetric BMD [68].

Conclusions

Gonadal failure (or even a delay of sex steroid secretion) during the period when the skeleton acquires 50% of its bone mineral is a major health problem, potentially with consequences into old age. In this regard, age-associated osteoporosis may in part be considered a pediatric disease. To date, most studies have focused only on issues such as the development of secondary sex characteristics, the acquisition of optimal height and body distribution. The classical DXA tool that is used to measure skeletal changes in adults does not appropriately differentiate the dramatic changes in trabecular and cortical compartments that occur during peak bone mass acquisition. Thus, many challenges remain for the everyday clinician.

Although evidence to allow firm recommendations is still lacking, it would seem that replacement therapy should aim to mimic sex steroid levels as closely as possible to those in the context of normal sex steroid secretion. Studies that advocate postponing sex steroid replacement in TS patients in order to increase height or interference with aromatization of androgens in delayed puberty should also document that peak bone mass acquisition in the different skeletal compartments is not blunted by this approach.

Acknowledgments

D. Vanderschueren and S. Boonen are senior clinical investigators of the Fund for Scientific Research, Flanders, Belgium (FWO-Vlaanderen). This review was supported by grant G.0171.03 from the Fund for Scientific Research, Flanders, Belgium to S. Boonen. S. Boonen is holder of the Leuven University Chair in Metabolic Bone Diseases.

References

1 Saggese G, Baroncelli GI, Bertelloni S: Puberty and bone development. Best Pract Res Clin Endocrinol Metab 2002;16:53–64.
2 Soyka LA, Fairfield WP, Klibanski A: Clinical review 117: Hormonal determinants and disorders of peak bone mass in children. J Clin Endocrinol Metab 2000;85:3951–3963.
3 Lu PW, Cowell CT, LLoyd-Jones SA, Briody JN, Howman-Giles R: Volumetric bone mineral density in normal subjects, aged 5–27 years. J Clin Endocrinol Metab 1996;81:1586–1590.
4 Seeman E: Pathogenesis of bone fragility in women and men. Lancet 2002;359:1841–1850.
5 Bass S, Delmas PD, Pearce G, Hendrich E, Tabensky A, Seeman E: The differing tempo of growth in bone size, mass, and density in girls is region-specific. J Clin Invest 1999;104:795–804.
6 Riggs BL, Khosla S, Melton LJ 3rd: The assembly of the adult skeleton during growth and maturation: implications for senile osteoporosis. J Clin Invest 1999;104:671–672.
7 Carter DR, Bouxsein ML, Marcus R: New approaches for interpreting projected bone densitometry data. J Bone Miner Res 1992;7:137–145.
8 Juul A: The effects of oestrogens on linear bone growth. Hum Reprod Update 2001;7:303–313.
9 Kim BT, Mosekilde L, Duan Y, Zhang XZ, Tornvig L, Thomsen JS, Seeman E: The structural and hormonal basis of sex differences in peak appendicular bone strength in rats. J Bone Miner Res 2003;18:150–155.
10 Turner RT, Wakley GK, Hannon KS: Differential effects of androgens on cortical bone histomorphometry in gonadectomized male and female rats. J Orthop Res 1990;8:612–617.
11 Riggs BL, Khosla S, Melton LJ 3rd: Sex steroids and the construction and conservation of the adult skeleton. Endocr Rev 2002;23:279–302.
12 Khosla S, Melton LJ 3rd, Riggs BL: Estrogen and the male skeleton. J Clin Endocrinol Metab 2002;87:1443–1450.
13 Vanderschueren D, Vandenput L, Boonen S, Lindberg MK, Bouillon R, Ohlsson C: Androgens and bone. Endocr Rev 2004;25:389–425.
14 Munoz-Torres M, Jodar E, Quesada M, Escobar-Jimenez F: Bone mass in androgen-insensitivity syndrome: Response to hormonal replacement therapy. Calcif Tissue Int 1995;57:94–96.
15 Soule SG, Conway G, Prelevic GM, Prentice M, Ginsburg J, Jacobs HS: Osteopenia as a feature of the androgen insensitivity syndrome. Clin Endocrinol 1995;43:671–675.
16 Mizunuma H, Soda M, Okano H, Kagami I, Miyamoto S, Ohsawa M, Ibuki Y: Changes in bone mineral density after orchidectomy and hormone replacement therapy in individuals with androgen insensitivity syndrome. Hum Reprod 1998;13:2816–2818.
17 Bertelloni S, Baroncelli GI, Federico G, Cappa M, Lala R, Saggese G: Altered bone mineral density in patients with complete androgen insensitivity syndrome. Horm Res 1998;50:309–314.
18 Marcus R, Leary D, Schneider DL, Shane E, Favus M, Quigley CA: The contribution of testosterone to skeletal development and maintenance: Lessons from the androgen insensitivity syndrome. J Clin Endocrinol Metab 2000;85:1032–1037.

19 Weissberger AJ, Ho KK: Activation of the somatotropic axis by testosterone in adult males: Evidence for the role of aromatization. J Clin Endocrinol Metab 1993;76:1407–1412.
20 Vanderschueren D, Boonen S, Ederveen AGH, De Coster R, Van Herck E, Moermans K, Vandenput L, Verstuyf A, Bouillon R: Skeletal effects of estrogen deficiency as induced by an aromatase inhibitor in an aged male rat model. Bone 2000;27:611–617.
21 Vandenput L, Swinnen JV, Van Herck E, Verstuyf A, Boonen S, Bouillon R, Vanderschueren D: The estrogen receptor ligand ICI 182,780 does not impair the bone-sparing effects of testosterone in the young orchidectomized rat model. Calcif Tissue Int 2002;70:170–175.
22 Keenan BS, Richards GE, Ponder SW, Dallas JS, Nagamani M, Smith ER: Androgen-stimulated pubertal growth: The effects of testosterone and dihydrotestosterone on growth hormone and insulin-like growth factor-I in the treatment of short stature and delayed puberty. J Clin Endocrinol Metab 1993;76:996–1001.
23 Klein KO, Baron J, Colli MJ, McDonnell DP, Cutler GB Jr: Estrogen levels in childhood determined by an ultrasensitive recombinant cell bioassay. J Clin Invest 1994;94:2475–2480.
24 Labrie F, Belanger A, Cusan L, Gomez J-L, Candas B: Marked decline in serum concentrations of adrenal C19 sex steroid precursors and conjugated androgen metabolites during aging. Endocrinology 1997;82:2396–2402.
25 Zborowski JV, Cauley JA, Talbott EO, Guzick DS, Winters SJ: Bone mineral density, androgens, and the polycystic ovary: The complex and controversial issue of androgenic influence in female bone. J Clin Endocrinol Metab 2000;85:3496–3506.
26 Buchanan JR, Hospodar P, Myers C, Leuenberger P, Demers LM: Effect of excess endogenous androgens on bone density in young women. J Clin Endocrinol Metab 1988;67:937–943.
27 Dagogo-Jack S, al-Ali N, Qurttom M: Augmentation of bone mineral density in hirsute women. J Clin Endocrinol Metab 1997;82:2821–2825.
28 Finkelstein JS, Neer RM, Biller BM, Crawford JD, Klibanski A: Osteopenia in men with a history of delayed puberty. N Engl J Med 1992;326:600–604.
29 Bertelloni S, Baroncelli GI, Battini R, Perri G, Saggese G: Short-term effects of testosterone treatment on reduced bone density in boys with constitutional delay of puberty. J Bone Miner Res 1995;10:1488–1495.
30 Finkelstein JS, Klibanski A, Neer RM: A longitudinal evaluation of bone mineral density in adult men with histories of delayed puberty. J Clin Endocrinol Metab 1996;81:1152–1155.
31 Moreira-Andres MN, Canizo FJ, de la Cruz FJ, Gomez-de la Camara A, Hawkins FG: Bone mineral status in prepubertal children with constitutional delay of growth and puberty. Eur J Endocrinol 1998;139:271–275.
32 Bertelloni S, Baroncelli GI, Ferdeghini M, Perri G, Saggese G: Normal volumetric bone mineral density and bone turnover in young men with histories of constitutional delay of puberty. J Clin Endocrinol Metab 1998;83:4280–4283.
33 Finkelstein JS, Klibanski A, Neer RM: Evaluation of lumber spine bone mineral density (BMD) using dual energy X-ray absorptiometry (DXA) in 21 young men with histories of constitutionally-delayed puberty. J Clin Endocrinol Metab 1999;84:3400–3401;author reply 3403–3404.
34 Finkelstein JS, Klibanski A, Neer RM, Greenspan SL, Rosenthal DI, Crowley WF Jr: Osteoporosis in men with idiopathic hypogonadotropic hypogonadism. Ann Intern Med 1987;106:354–361.
35 Finkelstein JS, Klibanski A, Neer RM, Doppelt SH, Rosenthal DI, Segre GV, Crowley WF Jr: Increases in bone density during treatment of men with idiopathic hypogonadotropic hypogonadism. J Clin Endocrinol Metab 1989;69:776–783.
36 Guo C-Y, Jones TH, Eastell R: Treatment of isolated hypogonadotropic hypogonadism effect on bone mineral density and bone turnover. J Clin Endocrinol Metab 1997;82:658–665.
37 Greenspan SL, Neer RM, Ridgway EC, Klibanski A: Osteoporosis in men with hyperprolactinemic hypogonadism. Ann Intern Med 1986;104:777–782.
38 Greenspan SL, Oppenheim DS, Klibanski A: Importance of gonadal steroids to bone mass in men with hyperprolactinemic hypogonadism. Ann Intern Med 1989;110:526–531.
39 Luisetto G, Mastrogiacomo I, Bonanni G, Pozzan G, Botteon S, Tizian L, Galuppo P: Bone mass and mineral metabolism in Klinefelter's syndrome. Osteoporosis Int 1995;5:455–461.
40 Smith DAS, Walker MS: Changes in plasma steroids and bone density in Klinefelter's syndrome. Calcif Tissue Res 1977;22:225–228.

41 Foresta C, Ruzza G, Mioni R, Meneghello A, Baccichetti C: Testosterone and bone loss in Klinefelter syndrome. Horm Metab Res 1983;15:56–57.
42 Horowitz M, Wishart JM, O'Loughlin PD, Morris HA, Need AG, Nordin BEC: Osteoporosis and Klinefelter's syndrome. Clin Endocrinol 1992;36:113–118.
43 Wong FH, Pun KK, Wang C: Loss of bone mass in patients with Klinefelter's syndrome despite sufficient testosterone replacement. Osteoporosis Int 1993;3:3–7.
44 van den Bergh JP, Hermus AR, Spruyt AI, Sweep CG, Corstens FH, Smals AG: Bone mineral density and quantitative ultrasound parameters in patients with Klinefelter's syndrome after long-term testosterone substitution. Osteoporosis Int 2001;12:55–62.
45 Batch J: Turner syndrome in childhood and adolescence. Best Pract Res Clin Endocrinol Metab 2002;16:465–482.
46 Clement-Jones M, Schiller S, Rao E, Blaschke RJ, Zuniga A, Zeller R, Robson SC, Binder G, Glass I, Strachan T, Lindsay S, Rappold GA: The short stature homeobox gene SHOX is involved in skeletal abnormalities in Turner syndrome. Hum Mol Genet 2000;9:695–702.
47 Davies MC, Gulekli B, Jacobs HS: Osteoporosis in Turner's syndrome and other forms of primary amenorrhoea. Clin Endocrinol (Oxf) 1995;43:741–746.
48 Shaw NJ, Rehan VK, Husain S, Marshall T, Smith CS: Bone mineral density in Turner's syndrome: A longitudinal study. Clin Endocrinol (Oxf) 1997;47:367–370.
49 Ross JL, Long LM, Feuillan P, Cassorla F, Cutler GB Jr: Normal bone density of the wrist and spine and increased wrist fractures in girls with Turner's syndrome. J Clin Endocrinol Metab 1991;73:355–359.
50 Bertelloni S, Cinquanta L, Baroncelli GI, Simi P, Rossi S, Saggese G: Volumetric bone mineral density in young women with Turner's syndrome treated with estrogens or estrogens plus growth hormone. Horm Res 2000;53:72–76.
51 Bechtold S, Rauch F, Noelle V, Donhauser S, Neu CM, Schoenau E, Schwarz HP: Musculoskeletal analyses of the forearm in young women with Turner syndrome: A study using peripheral quantitative computed tomography. J Clin Endocrinol Metab 2001;86:5819–5823.
52 Sas TC, de Muinck Keizer-Schrama SM, Stijnen T, van Teunenbroek A, van Leeuwen WJ, Asarfi A, van Rijn RR, Drop SL, Dutch Advisory Group on Growth Hormone: Bone mineral density assessed by phalangeal radiographic absorptiometry before and during long-term growth hormone treatment in girls with Turner's syndrome participating in a randomized dose-response study. Pediatr Res 2001;50:417–422.
53 Gravholt CH, Lauridsen AL, Brixen K, Mosekilde L, Heickendorff L, Christiansen JS: Marked disproportionality in bone size and mineral, and distinct abnormalities in bone markers and calcitropic hormones in adult turner syndrome: A cross-sectional study. J Clin Endocrinol Metab 2002;87:2798–2808.
54 Bakalov VK, Axelrod L, Baron J, Hanton L, Nelson LM, Reynolds JC, Hill S, Troendle J, Bondy CA: Selective reduction in cortical bone mineral density in turner syndrome independent of ovarian hormone deficiency. J Clin Endocrinol Metab 2003;88:5717–5722.
55 Bakalov VK, Chen ML, Baron J, Hanton LB, Reynolds JC, Stratakis CA, Axelrod LE, Bondy CA: Bone mineral density and fractures in Turner syndrome. Am J Med 2003;115:259–264.
56 Hogler W, Briody J, Moore B, Garnett S, Lu PW, Cowell CT: Importance of estrogen on bone health in Turner syndrome: A cross-sectional and longitudinal study using dual-energy X-ray absorptiometry. J Clin Endocrinol Metab 2004;89:193–199.
57 Landin-Wilhelmsen K, Bryman I, Windh M, Wilhelmsen L: Osteoporosis and fractures in Turner syndrome-importance of growth promoting and oestrogen therapy. Clin Endocrinol (Oxf) 1999;51:497–502.
58 Gravholt CH, Vestergaard P, Hermann AP, Mosekilde L, Brixen K, Christiansen JS: Increased fracture rates in Turner's syndrome: A nationwide questionnaire survey. Clin Endocrinol (Oxf) 2003;59:89–96.
59 Mauras N, Haymond MW, Darmaun D, Vieira NE, Abrams SA, Yergey AL: Calcium and protein kinetics in prepubertal boys: Positive effects of testosterone. J Clin Invest 1994;93:1014–1019.
60 van Pareren YK, de Muinck Keizer-Schrama SM, Stijnen T, Sas TC, Jansen M, Otten BJ, Hoorweg-Nijman JJ, Vulsma T, Stokvis-Brantsma WH, Rouwe CW, Reeser HM, Gerver WJ, Gosen JJ, Rongen-Westerlaken C, Drop SL: Final height in girls with turner syndrome after long-term growth

hormone treatment in three dosages and low dose estrogens. J Clin Endocrinol Metab 2003; 88:1119–1125.
61 Nilsson KO, Albertsson-Wikland K, Alm J, Aronson S, Gustafsson J, Hagenas L, Hager A, Ivarsson SA, Karlberg J, Kristrom B, Marcus C, Moell C, Ritzen M, Tuvemo T, Wattsgard C, Westgren U, Westphal O, Aman J: Improved final height in girls with Turner's syndrome treated with growth hormone and oxandrolone. J Clin Endocrinol Metab 1996;81:635–640.
62 Khastgir G, Studd JW, Fox SW, Jones J, Alaghband-Zadeh J, Chow JW: A longitudinal study of the effect of subcutaneous estrogen replacement on bone in young women with Turner's syndrome. J Bone Miner Res 2003;18:925–932.
63 Pozo J, Argente J: Ascertainment and treatment of delayed puberty. Horm Res 2003;60(suppl 3): 35–48.
64 Wickman S, Kajantie E, Dunkel L: Effects of suppression of estrogen action by the p450 aromatase inhibitor letrozole on bone mineral density and bone turnover in pubertal boys. J Clin Endocrinol Metab 2003;88:3785–3793.
65 Schroor EJ, van Weissenbruch MM, Knibbe P, Delemarre-van de Waal HA: The effect of prolonged administration of an anabolic steroid (oxandrolone) on growth in boys with constitutionally delayed growth and puberty. Eur J Pediatr 1995;154:953–957.
66 Lampit M, Hochberg Z: Androgen therapy in constitutional delay of growth. Horm Res 2003;59:270–275.
67 Wickman S, Sipila I, Ankarberg-Lindgren C, Norjavaara E, Dunkel L: A specific aromatase inhibitor and potential increase in adult height in boys with delayed puberty: a randomised controlled trial. Lancet 2001;357:1743–1748.
68 Vanderschueren D, Van Herck E, Nijs J, Ederveen AG, De Coster R, Bouillon R: Aromatase inhibition impairs skeletal modeling and decreases bone mineral density in growing male rats. Endocrinology 1997;138:2301–2307.

Dirk Vanderschueren, MD, PhD
Laboratory for Experimental Medicine and Endocrinology
Katholieke Universiteit Leuven, Campus Gasthuisberg
Onderwijs & Navorsing, Herestraat 49, BE–3000 Leuven (Belgium)
Tel. +32 16 345970, Fax +32 16 345934, E-Mail dirk.vanderschueren@uz.kuleuven.ac.be

Delemarre-van de Waal HA (ed): Abnormalities in Puberty. Scientific and Clinical Advances.
Endocr Dev. Basel, Karger, 2005, vol 8, pp 166–175

Present and Future Options for the Preservation of Fertility in Female Adolescents with Cancer

C.C.M. Beerendonk, D.D.M. Braat

Department of Obstetrics and Gynaecology,
University Medical Centre St Radboud, Nijmegen, The Netherlands

Abstract

Fertility and sexuality are important aspects in the quality of life of long-term survivors of cancer. Adolescents in particular are in a very vulnerable period of their lives with respect to future fertility and sexuality. Special attention should be paid to preserve their fertility whenever possible. The gonadotoxic effect of chemotherapy is largely drug- and dose-dependent and is related to age. The effect of radiotherapy is also dependent on dose and age and on the radiation therapy field. The prepubertal ovary is the least susceptible to gonadotoxicity. Ablative regimens for stem cell transplantation have an extremely high risk of ovarian failure. Alternative chemotherapy protocols can reduce long-term gonadotoxicity. Alkylating agents impose the highest risk in causing ovarian failure and should be avoided whenever possible. Up to now, the results of gonadoprotective hormonal therapy have been disappointing and contradictory. Transposition of the ovaries should be considered in each case of planned pelvic or whole body irradiation, where ovarian involvement is unlikely and chemotherapy not necessary. Cryopreservation of preimplantation embryos will seldom be possible in female adolescents due to the lack of a stable relationship with a male partner. Cryopreservation of mature and immature oocytes (necessitating in vitro maturation) is still assumed not to be safe for the offspring. Cryopreservation and transplantation of ovarian tissue seems to be the most promising way of future fertility preservation in female adolescents. At present, it is in its early experimental stage. Its safety and possibilities for fertility preservation in humans are not proven as yet. Additionally, technical and ethical issues need to be addressed. The counseling of female adolescents who are facing the threat of cancer needs careful consideration with regards to the psychosocial impact of the treatment and its consequences. Special attention should be paid to aspects of future quality of life, in particular: fertility and sexuality.

As long-term survival of cancer is improving, the awareness of long-term consequences of cancer therapy is growing. In general, quality of life after cancer therapy is widely researched. Fertility and sexuality are important aspects within this field. Especially in cases of cancer therapy in adolescence care should be taken for the (future) endocrine, sexual, and fertility consequences. Adolescents are in a particular vulnerable period of their lives with many new challenges with regards to their psychosocial development (sexual maturation, marriage, employment, etc.). They deserve special attention when cancer threatens their lives. The overall incidence of cancer in 15- to 19-year-olds is approximately 50% higher than the incidence of cancer in children less than 15 years of age [1]. Although the survival rates have improved during recent years, they have not kept pace with the survival rates in younger patients. The participation rate alone in clinical trials in this age group is very low in comparison with the children and adult groups. The cause of this so-called adolescent and young adult gap is largely unknown and multifactorial. It appears that adolescents are not considered a separate group, but squeezed in between pediatric and adult oncological care. As this problem has been identified already many years ago, it is only recently that special attention is paid to the consequences.

In this chapter, we will focus on the possibilities of preservation of fertility in female adolescents with cancer. Apart from the clinical aspects, ethical issues will be considered. Furthermore, the counseling of these patients and their parents with regard to their future fertility will be addressed.

Effects of Chemotherapy and Radiotherapy on Female Fertility

Normally, at birth around 1,000,000 oocytes are present. This number declines to 250,000 at menarche, after which only 400–500 eggs will eventually ovulate. At the age of 37, the number of eggs declines even faster (for unknown reasons), resulting in a significant impairment of fertility. At a mean age of 52 (around 1,000 eggs left), normal menopause takes place. Normal fertility already appears to be decreased 5–10 years before menopause, also in case of regular cycles. The first sign of this decrease in fertility is a higher follicle-stimulating hormone (FSH) level in the early follicular phase (day 1–3) of the menstrual cycle. Criteria for elevated FSH levels differ per clinic, but often levels >10 or >15 IU/l are considered to be abnormal, whereas an FSH level >40 IU/l is considered to be menopausal. Chemotherapy and radiotherapy will damage the ovary. In contrast to the situation in men, there is no clear separation in a hormonal and a fertility effect of ovarian dysfunction. The gonadotoxic effects of chemotherapy in females are drug- and dose-dependent (cumulative) and are related to the age at the time of treatment. The smaller the dose, the later the age ovarian failure occurs. Alkylating agents (cyclophosphamide, *L*-phenylalanine mustard, chlorambucil, busulfan) are deleterious for the ovarian function. They interact with DNA and thus damage ovarian tissue permanently. It appears that not only follicular maturation is impaired but that primordial follicles are also depleted. Methotrexate, 5-fluorouracil, etoposide and doxorubicin do not induce permanent ovarian failure [2]. Induction of apoptosis in pre-granulosa cells appears to be the primary way of action of chemotherapy-induced follicle loss. The prepubertal and adolescent ovary is less susceptible to alkylkating chemotherapy than the ovaries of women in their late twenties and beyond [3, 4].

The response of the ovaries to radiation is also dependent on dose and age. An ovarian dose of 4 Gy leads to sterility in 30% of young women and in 100% of women over age 40. Recently, Wallace et al. [5] estimated the LD_{50} of the human oocyte to be <2 Gy. According to his mathematical model, the age of menopause can be predicted for a given dose of radiotherapy.

The presence of normal reproductive parameters after chemotherapy and/or radiotherapy does not imply that no ovarian damage has occurred. Partial loss of primordial follicles can lead to premature ovarian failure (POF) as a delayed reaction to treatment. Byrne et al. [6] interviewed 1,067 women after treatment for cancer during childhood and adolescence. They found relative risks of POF during the early twenties of 9.2 after alkylating agents alone and of 3.7 after radiotherapy alone. Abdominal radiotherapy in combination with alkylating agents increased the risk of POF 27-fold. By the age of 31, 42% had reached menopause compared with 5% for controls. Larsen et al. [7] evaluated 100 female childhood cancer survivors who had a median age of 25.7 years at study entry. Seventeen of these women had already reached menopause. The investigators performed multiple linear regression analysis to predict the total antral follicle number per ovary. It showed a reduced number with ovarian irradiation, alkylating chemotherapy, older age at diagnosis and longer time period off treatment. Consequently, childhood and adolescent cancer survivors with spontaneous cycles are still at risk for POF and may have a small fertility window.

Pelvic irradiation can lead to impaired uterine growth in premenarchal girls and failure of uterine expansion during pregnancy, leading to miscarriages and premature births [8]. The radiation effect on the uterus is unpredictable, but higher doses are more likely to be associated with vascular and uterine damage [9]. One cohort study of female survivors of childhood cancer (treated with either chemo- and/or radiotherapy) has shown no significant differences in pregnancy outcome by treatment. A higher, but not statistically significant, risk of miscarriage was present among women whose ovaries were in the radiation therapy field. Furthermore, the offspring of women who received pelvic irradiation are at risk for low birth weight [10].

Effects of Stem Cell Transplantation on Female Fertility

Stem cell transplantation (SCT) is the treatment of choice in most cases of hematological malignancies at young age. The conditioning regimens used for SCT include high-dose chemotherapy, usually combined with total body irradiation (TBI). These ablative regimens have an extremely high risk for ovarian failure, even in girls treated prepubertally [11]. In 20–65% of girls who receive SCT with high-dose chemotherapy and TBI before puberty, menarche and the onset of puberty occur spontaneously [11–14]. Girls who receive SCT after their menarche and with an ablative conditioning regimen almost all develop amenorrhoea [11, 14]. Basal FSH is elevated in all of these girls and LH is elevated in most. If the onset of puberty is delayed, hormonal therapy (HT) may be necessary [13]. Conditioning with chemotherapy alone and SCT before menarche lead to the best chance of recovery of ovarian function [11]. In a study by Sanders et al. [4], in all women treated with high-dose cyclophosphamide alone, before 26 years of age, recovery of ovarian function occurred. As addressed above already, however, this does not exclude an early menopause.

Androgen levels are lower after SCT than after chemotherapy or in healthy controls. Subnormal androgen production might be one factor of importance behind the problems in puberty development and in adult sex life after SCT [14].

Twenty to 50% of patients develop chronic graft vs. host disease (GVHD) after allogeneic SCT. The role of GVHD in fertility disorders, sexual dysfunction and pregnancy has to be determined. Marks et al. [15] found that 5 of 6 patients with GVHD had sexual dysfunction.

Present and Future Options for Gonadoprotection in Case of Chemotherapy

The use of alternative chemotherapy protocols with or without additive radiotherapy can reduce long-term gonadotoxicity. Alkylating agents should be avoided when possible as they impose the highest risk in causing ovarian failure [2]. Several strategies have been proposed to suppress the gonadostat: gonadotropin-releasing hormone agonists, oral contraceptive pills, medroxyprogesterone acetate. A protective effect was expected as dividing cells are much more sensitive to chemotherapeutics than resting cells. However, study results are contradictory and as yet no randomized controlled trials with sufficient power have been performed. Therefore, we agree with Sonmezer and Oktay [16] that in the absence of convincing evidence, we do not recommend ovarian suppression as an effective means of fertility preservation. Whenever ovarian suppression is considered, it should only be applied within the setup of a randomized controlled trial.

When the molecular and genetic framework of chemotherapy-induced germ cell death is identified, apoptotic inhibitors may be developed in the future. Genetic manipulation may also play a future role in reducing the damage imposed by chemotherapeutics [17].

Present and Future Options for Gonadoprotection in Case of Radiotherapy

Hormonal suppression of the gonadostat by MPA or GnRH-a appears to radiosensitize the ovaries in rats instead of protecting them [18, 19]. The radiation doses used with standard pelvic irradiation will induce ovarian failure. To reduce the dose in adolescents and young women, ovarian transposition should be performed before pelvic irradiation. Of course, this can only be considered when the risk of ovarian involvement is negligible. When abdomino-pelvic surgery is not planned, ovarian transposition can best be performed laparoscopically just before the start of radiation therapy because of the risk of spontaneous migration back to the original position [17]. The optimal way to preserve ovarian reserve is lateral transposition of the ovaries above the iliac crest in contrast to medial transposition behind the uterus. An alternative to ovarian transposition before pelvic irradiation is shielding of the ovaries by lead slabs during radiotherapy [20]. Both techniques are only partially successful [21]. Consequently, the value of ovarian transposition or shielding in women over 40 years of age is limited because lower irradiation doses already cause ovarian failure. In a recent experiment, heterotopic transposition was undertaken of an intact ovary with vascular anastomosis in a patient with cervical cancer [Hilders et al., COBRA-dagen, Noordwijkerhout, The Netherlands, 2004]. The functional result of this procedure is not yet known.

Present and Future Options for Gonadoprotection in Case of Stem Cell Transplantation

By using a less aggressive, non-ablative approach for conditioning before SCT (high-dose melfalan) in cases of Hodgkin's disease and non-Hodgkin's lymphoma, a substantial part of fertility can be preserved. This non-ablative approach has been as effective as the more aggressive regimens in treating the malignancy [22]. It was additionally shown that fractionated TBI is less toxic to the ovaries than single-dose TBI, even in higher doses [11]. As far as known to us, no studies have been performed as yet to investigate the effect of suppression of GVHD on future gonadal function.

Other Present and Future Options for Fertility Preservation

Cryopreservation of embryos is a standard procedure in established IVF programs. This procedure can also be offered as fertility preservation in case of cancer therapy. After egg collection all oocytes are inseminated and subsequently all fertilized eggs are cryopreserved. These embryos might be thawed and transferred into the uterus in later life (after recovering from cancer). This procedure can only be performed in case of a stable relationship, because only fertilized eggs (embryos) can be frozen. Although sometimes it is suggested to use donor sperm, this isn't a realistic option for most women. It is difficult to predict the chances of success, in normal IVF procedures the pregnancy rate per embryo transfer of frozen embryos is around 10%. Another factor is that the patient should be physically and psychologically able to undergo hormonal stimulation and follicular puncture, and she should have the time to postpone cancer treatment. In this treatment, after freezing, the normal procedures take place (as in freezing in routine IVF procedures) with respect to informed consent and destination of the embryos in case one or both partners die. Consequently, IVF with freezing all embryos will seldom be the method of choice in adolescents.

Cryopreservation of mature oocytes is still experimental and very debatable because of low pregnancy rates per thawed oocyte (about 1.5%) and worries about the safety of the method for the offspring. In 1986, the first pregnancy by this method was reported [23]. Since then 2 major congenital abnormalities were reported in only 32 pregnancies [16]. This treatment also requires time for ovarian stimulation and follicle aspiration, and can therefore only take place if there is time to postpone cancer treatment.

It is possible to collect and freeze immature oocytes [24]. Immature frozen-thawed oocytes need in vitro maturation. During this process spindle and chromosome abnormalities have been reported. Only a few pregnancies using frozen-thawed immature oocytes have been reported thus far [16].

Up to now, cryopreservation and transplantation of ovarian tissue seems to be the most promising way of fertility preservation in adolescents. Although this procedure is now offered worldwide in many clinics, this too is still an experimental procedure. The limiting factor in cryopreservation of a whole human ovary is the rate of uniform penetration with cryoprotectants. At present, small ovarian cortical strips have been cryopreserved successfully. After transplantation of these frozen-thawed ovarian cortical strips, up to two-thirds of follicles are lost due to initial ischemia. In animals, pregnancies and deliveries have been reported after ovarian cryopreservation and transplantation. In humans, resumption of endocrine activity has been demonstrated and the first embryo has been obtained after subcutaneous transplantation of frozen-thawed ovarian tissue [25]. The first human pregnancy has been reported on June 30, 2004 by Professor Donnez (Brussels, Belgium). Because of the possibility of ovarian metastases and therefore the risk of reintroducing the cancer, transplantation of ovarian tissue in case of hematological cancers like leukemia, Burkitt's lymphoma, some breast and colon cancers and neuroblastoma cases should not be performed [26–28].

Endocrine activity appears to be better after heterotopic transplantation (maximum 3 years) than after orthotopic transplantation (maximum 9 months). However, these conclusions are all based on case-reports and not on large prospective trials. Xenografting of human ovarian tissue to immunodeficient mice is an ideal model to study different aspects of human ovarian tissue autotransplantation. In case of a high probability of ovarian metastatic disease, xenografting may be considered as a means to utilize banked ovarian tissue in the future. This technique, however, raises many technical and ethical concerns.

Alternatives

As gonadotoxicity by chemotherapy and radiotherapy is less in adolescents, one can also consider a wait and see policy, particularly in a case of high-risk ovarian involvement. In that case, the woman should be aware of the high risk of premature ovarian failure although ovarian function appears to be restored shortly after cancer therapy. Another alternative is oocyte donation in case of ovarian failure after cancer treatment. This is a very successful established treatment option with potentially high pregnancy rates (up to 60% per embryo transfer). The pregnancy rate is predominantly related to the age of the egg donor. The option of adoption should also be discussed with these patients.

Ethical Considerations and Counselling

Patients suffering from cancer and their parents should be informed about the (im)possibilities of preservation of fertility. Although many procedures are possible, they still all are experimental. This should be discussed with the patients and their parents. They also should be carefully informed about the risks and the uncertainties of the procedures as well as the uncertainties of its use in the future. In case of freezing ovarian tissue the patient should sign an informed consent. She should know that there is a chance that it might never be used [29].

Ideally, the patient should be referred to a gynecologist who is familiar with these procedures and with the potential risks and complications.

Conclusions

Attention for preservation of fertility in female adolescents with cancer is important because long-term survival of cancer is increasing and the ability of procreation represents an important aspect of the quality of life. These young women are also in a particular vulnerable period of their lives with already many uncertainties with regards to their psychosocial development.

Pharmacological protection up to now has been very disappointing. Less-aggressive chemotherapy regimens with less risk of ovarian failure need to be developed. When pelvic or total body irradiation is necessary and ovarian involvement is unlikely, laparoscopic ovarian transposition should be considered shortly before the start of irradiation.

In the future, ovarian cryopreservation and transplantation are the most promising procedures for fertility preservation in female adolescents with cancer. Up to now it still is an experimental treatment of which the future possibilities can not be overseen as yet. Many technical and ethical issues need to be addressed. In counseling these young women, all of these aspects need to be considered. Alternatives such as oocyte donation, adoption or acceptance of being unable to have children should also be mentioned.

References

1 Bleyer WA: Overview: Cancer in older adolescents and young adults: Epidemiology, diagnosis, treatment, survival, and importance of clinical trials. Med Pediatr Oncol 2002;38:1–10.

2 Meirow D, Nugent D: The effects of radiotherapy and chemotherapy on female reproduction. Hum Reprod Update 2001;7:535–543.

3 Siris ES, Leventhal BG, Vaitukaitis JL: Effects of childhood leukaemia and chemotherapy on puberty and reproductive function in girls. N Engl J Med 1976;294:1143–1150.

4 Sanders JE, Buckner CD, Amos D, Levy W, Appelbaum FR, Doney K, Storb R, Sullivan KM, Witherspoon RP, Thomas ED: Ovarian function following marrow transplantation for aplastic anemia or leukemia. J Clin Oncol 1988;6:813–818.

5 Wallace WHB, Thomson AB, Kelsey TW: The radiosensitivity of the human oocyte. Hum Reprod 2003;18:117–121.

6 Byrne J, Fears TR, Gail MH, Pee D, Connelly RR, Austin DF, Holmes GF, Holmes FF, Latourette HB, Meigs JW, Strong LC, Myers MH, Mulvihill JJ: Early menopause in long-term survivors of cancer during adolescence. Am J Obstet Gynecol 1992;166:788–793.
7 Larsen EC, Muller J, Schmiegelow K, Rechtnitzer C, Andersen AN: Reduced ovarian function in long-term survivors of radiation- and chemotherapy-treated childhood cancer. J Clin Endocrinol Metab 2003;88:5307–5314.
8 Ogilvy-Stuart AL, Shalet SM: Effect of radiation on the human reproductive system. Environ Health Perspect 1993;101(suppl 2):109–116.
9 Critchley HO, Bath LE, Wallace WH: Radiation damage to the uterus – review of the effects of treatment of childhood cancer. Hum Fertil (Camb) 2002;5:61–66.
10 Green DM, Whitton JA, Stovall M, Mertens AC, Donaldson SS, Ruymann FB, Pendergrass TW, Robison LL: Pregnancy outcome of female survivors of childhood cancer: A report from the Childhood Cancer Survivor Study. Am J Obstet Gynecol 2002;187:1070–1080.
11 Thibaud E, Rodriguez-Macias K, Trivin C, Esperou H, Michon J, Brauner R: Ovarian function after bone marrow transplantation during childhood. Bone Marrow Transplant 1998;21:287–290.
12 Bakker B, Massa GG, Oostdijk W, Van Weel-Sipman MH, Vossen JM, Wit JM: Pubertal development and growth after total-body irradiation and bone marrow transplantation for haematological malignancies. Eur J Pediatr 2000;159:31–37.
13 Mayer EI, Dopfer RE, Klingebiel T, Scheel-Walter H, Ranke MB, Niethammer D: Longitudinal gonadal function after bone marrow transplantation for acute lymphoblastic leukemia during childhood. Pediatr Transplant 1999;3:38–44.
14 Hovi L, Tapanainen P, Saarinen-Pihkala UM, Siimes MA: Impaired androgen production in female adolescents and young adults after total body irradiation prior to BMT in childhood. Bone Marrow Transplant 1997;20:561–565.
15 Marks DI, Friedman SH, Delli Carpini L, Nezu CM, Nezu AM: A prospective study of the effects of high-dose chemotherapy and bone marrow transplantation on sexual function in the first year after transplant. Bone Marrow Transplant 1997;19:819–822.
16 Sonmezer M, Oktay K: Fertility preservation in female patients. Hum Reprod Update 2004;10: 251–266.
17 Falcone T, Attaran M, Bedaiwy MA, Goldberg JM: Ovarian function preservation in the cancer patient. Fertil Steril 2004;81:243–257.
18 Jarrell J, YoungLai EV, McMahon A, Barr R, O'Connell G, Belbec L: The effect of medroxyprogesterone acetate (Provera) on ovarian radiosensitivity. Am J Obstet Gynecol 1989;160: 990–994.
19 Jarrell JF, McMahon A, Barr RD, YoungLai EV: The agonist (d-leu-6,des-gly-10)-LHRH-ethylamide does not protect the fecundity of rats exposed to high dose unilateral ovarian irradiation. Reprod Toxicol 1991;5:385–388.
20 Treissman MJ, Miller D, McComb PF: Laparoscopic lateral ovarian transposition. Fertil Steril 1996;65:1229–1231.
21 Damewood MD, Grochow LB: Prospects for fertility after chemotherapy or radiation for neoplastic disease. Fertil Steril 1986;45:443–459.
22 Jackson GH, Wood A, Taylor PR, Lennard AL, Lucraft H, Heppleston A, Robinson P, Moore J, Proctor SJ: Early high dose chemotherapy intensification with autologous bone marrow transplantation in lymphoma associated with retention of fertility and normal pregnancies in females. Leuk Lymphoma 1997;28:127–132.
23 Chen C: Pregnancy after human oocyte cryopreservation. Lancet 1986;327:884–886.
24 Tucker MJ, Wright G, Morton PC, Massey JB: Birth after cryopreservation of immature oocytes with subsequent in vitro maturation. Fertil Steril 1998;70:578–579.
25 Oktay K, Buyuk E, Veeck L, Zaninovic N, Xu K, Takeuchi T, Opsahl M, Rosenwaks Z: Embryo development after heterotopic transplantation of cryopreserved ovarian tissue. Lancet 2004; 363:1830.
26 Oktay K, Kan MT, Rosenwaks Z: Recent progress in oocyte and ovarian tissue cryopreservation and transplantation. Curr Opin Obstet Gynecol 2001;13:263–268.
27 McCarville MB, Hill DA, Miller BE, Pratt CB: Secondary ovarian neoplasms in children: Imaging features with histopathologic correlation. Pediatr Radiol 2001;31:358–364.

28 Yada-Hashimoto N, Yamamoto T, Kamiura S, Seino H, Ohira H, Sawai K, Kimura T, Saji F: Metastatic ovarian tumors: A review of 64 cases. Gynaecol Oncol 2003;89:314–317.
29 Hilhorst JA, Braat DDM, Goverde HJ, Ten Have HA: Cryopreservation of ovarian tissue; now is the time for ethical considerations. Ned Tijdschr Geneeskd 2000;144:695–698.

Dr. C.C.M. Beerendonk
UMCN St Radboud, Department of Obstetrics and Gynaecology
415, PO Box 9101, NL–6500 HB Nijmegen (The Netherlands)
Tel. +31 243613932, Fax +31 243541194, E-Mail C.Beerendonk@obgyn.umcn.nl

Author Index

Beerendonk, C.C.M. 166
Boonen, S. 150
Braat, D.D.M. 166

Claahsen-van der Grinten, H.L. 54

Delemarre-van de Waal, H.A. IX, 1, 15

Engelbregt, M.J.T. 15

Heger, S. 94
Hermus, A.R.M.M. 54
Homburg, R. 137

Johansson, T. 126
Jung, H. 81

Karges, B. 67

Ojeda, S.R. 81
Ong, K. 34
Otten, B.J. 54

Parent, A.-S. 81
Partsch, C.-J. 94

Ritzén, E.M. 126
Roux, N. de 67

Savage, M.O. VII
Sippell, W.G. 94
Stikkelbroeck, M.M.L. 54

Weissenbruch, M.M. van 15

Vandenput, L. 150
Vanderschueren, D. 150
Veening, M.A. 15

Subject Index

Androgens
aromatization into estrogen 154, 155
receptor-mediated effects on bone 155, 156
testosterone replacement therapy
delayed puberty 161
hypogonadism 159
Anorexia nervosa, puberty delay 7
Anosmin, mutation effects on puberty timing 5

Body mass index (BMI)
gonadotropin-releasing hormone agonist therapy outcomes 114
precocious puberty long-term follow-up in women 128
Bone mineral density (BMD)
bone development in puberty 150, 153
delayed puberty effects in males 157, 158
gonadal failure effects
females 159
males 158, 159
management 159, 160
gonadotropin-releasing hormone agonist therapy outcomes 114
polycystic ovary syndrome 157
sex steroid effects in puberty
androgen in males
aromatization into estrogen 154, 155
receptor-mediated effects 155, 156
females 157
growth hormone interactions 156
sexual dimorphism 151, 153

Cancer, *see* Fertility preservation, female cancer patients
Central precocious puberty, *see* Precocious puberty
Chemotherapy, *see* Fertility preservation, female cancer patients
Congenital adrenal hyperplasia (CAH)
antenatal management with glucocorticoids and long-term effects 40, 41, 57
clinical spectrum 55
fertility
females with 21-hydroxylase deficiency 58–60
males
child rates 60
secondary hypogonadotropism 62
testicular tumors 60–62
prevention of subfertility 62, 63
gene mutations 54
growth
adult height 57
prepuberty 56
pubertal growth 56, 57
precocious puberty 57, 58
puberty timing and progression 55, 56
Cortisol, *see* Glucocorticoids
Cyproterone acetate (CPA)
central precocious puberty management 104
polycystic ovary syndrome management in adolescence 145, 146

DAX-1, mutation effects on puberty timing 5, 6
DDT, endocrine disruption 8
Dehydroepiandrosterone sulfate (DHEAS)
clinical implications of glucocorticoid-induced excess
polycystic ovary syndrome 46, 47
premature pubarche 44, 45
low-birth-weight infant levels 42
small-for-gestational-age children levels 21, 22, 28, 42, 43
Delayed puberty
anorexia nervosa 7
bone mineral density effects in males 157, 158
long-term follow-up of women 133
management 161

Estrogen
androgen aromatization 154, 155
bone development role 151

Fertility preservation, female cancer patients
cancer incidence in adolescence 167
cryopreservation
fertilized oocytes 171
immature oocytes 171
mature oocytes 171
ovarian tissue preservation and transplantation 171–173
ethics and counseling 172, 173
gonadoprotection strategies
chemotherapy 169, 170, 173
radiation 170
stem cell transplantation 170, 171
oocyte donation 172
ovarian effects of cancer treatments
chemotherapy 167, 168
radiation 168, 169
stem cell transplantation 169
Fibroblast growth factor receptor 1 (FGFR1), gene mutations in Kallmann's syndrome 75
Finasteride, polycystic ovary syndrome management in adolescence 146
Flutamide, polycystic ovary syndrome management in adolescence 146
Follicle-stimulating hormone (FSH)
menopause onset 167
mutation effects on puberty timing 4
precocious puberty properties 9–11
receptor mutation effects on puberty timing 5
receptor structure 68, 69

Gli3, precocious puberty mechanisms in hypothalamic hamartoma 87, 88
Glucocorticoids
cortisol deficiency, *see* Congenital adrenal hyperplasia
exposure in perinatal period
antenatal therapy
congenital adrenal hyperplasia management 40, 41, 57
inhibition of development 35, 39
preterm infants 39, 40
cortisol deficiency in very-low-birth-weight infants in first few days of life 35, 36
cortisol excess in very-low-birth-weight infants after first few days of life
animal studies 37
dynamic responses 38, 39
fasting levels 37
methodological considerations 37, 38
11β-hydroxysteroid dehydrogenase activity in response to 41
Gonadoprotection, *see* Fertility preservation, female cancer patients
Gonadotropin-releasing hormone (GnRH)
agonists in central precocious puberty management
auxological effects 106
body mass index outcomes 114
bone mineral density outcomes 114
clinical, hormonal, and psychological effects 105, 106
final height effects 111–114
leuprorelin 104, 105
monitoring 108–110
overview 104

pituitary and gonadal function long-term effects 110, 111
prospects 115
psychosocial outcomes 115
randomized trials 105
side effects 106–108
triptorelin 104, 105
fetal testosterone effects on later secretion in females 16
precocious puberty properties 9–11
puberty onset role 1, 17
receptor
genotype-phenotype correlations in isolated hypogonadotropic hypogonadism 71, 72
mutation effects on puberty timing 6
structure 68–70
structure and function in isolated hypogonadotropic hypogonadism 69–71
sexual dimorphism 2
stimulation testing 109
GPR54
isolated hypogonadotropic hypogonadism defects 72–74
KISS-1 ligand 72, 73, 76
mutation effects on puberty timing 6
structure 68, 69
Graft-versus-host disease (GVHD), fertility effects in females 169
Growth hormone (GH)
sex steroid interactions in pubertal skeleton development 156
Turner's syndrome management 160

Height
congenital adrenal hyperplasia 57
gonadotropin-releasing hormone agonist therapy effects 111–114
intrauterine growth retardation effects 22, 23
precocious puberty long-term follow-up in women 127–129
21-Hydroxylase deficiency, *see* Congenital adrenal hyperplasia
11β-Hydroxysteroid dehydrogenase, activity in cortisol response 41
Hypogonadotropic hypogonadism, *see* Isolated hypogonadotropic hypogonadism
Hypothalamic hamartoma (HH)
anatomy 83–85
clinical features 82, 83
histology 81, 82
precocious puberty
etiology 82, 97
molecular mechanisms 85–89
prospects for study 89
sex differences 84, 85

Intrauterine growth retardation (IUGR)
dehydroepiandrosterone sulfate levels
clinical implications of glucocorticoid-induced excess
polycystic ovary syndrome 46, 47
premature pubarche 44, 45
low-birth-weight infants 42
small-for-gestational-age children 21, 22, 28, 42, 43
glucocorticoid exposure in perinatal period
antenatal therapy
congenital adrenal hyperplasia management 40, 41
inhibition of development 35, 39
preterm infants 39, 40
cortisol deficiency in very-low-birth-weight infants in first few days of life 35, 36
cortisol excess in very-low-birth-weight infants after first few days of life
animal studies 37
dynamic responses 38, 39
fasting levels 37
methodological considerations 37, 38
11β-hydroxysteroid dehydrogenase activity in response to 41
hypothalamic-pituitary-gonadotropin axis programming 16
metabolic syndrome risks 34, 35
polycystic ovary syndrome correlation 29

Intrauterine growth retardation (IUGR) (continued)
puberty timing effects
overview 7, 15–17
prospects for study 30
rat study of puberty onset
age at puberty onset 23
design 19, 20
ovarian development 24, 25–26, 28, 29
testicular development 26, 29, 30
weight and body composition 23, 24
small-for-gestational-age human study
clinical characteristics at birth 20
dehydroepiandrosterone sulfate levels 21, 22, 28
design 18, 19
linear growth 22, 23
sex differences 27
Isolated hypogonadotropic hypogonadism (IHH)
bone mineral density effects in males 158
gonadotropin-releasing hormone system defects 69–72
GPR54 mutations 73, 74

Kallmann's syndrome
clinical features 74
gene mutations 74, 75
KISS-1, GPR54 ligand 72, 73, 76
Klinefelter's syndrome, bone mineral density effects 158, 159

Leptin, puberty onset role 6, 7
Leuprorelin, central precocious puberty management 104, 105
Luteinizing hormone (LH)
mutation effects on puberty timing 4
precocious puberty properties 9–11
receptor
mutation effects on puberty timing 4, 5
structure 68, 69

Medroxyprogesterone acetate, central precocious puberty management 104
Menopause, onset 167
Mest, precocious puberty mechanisms in hypothalamic hamartoma 88
Metabolic syndrome, intrauterine growth retardation association 34, 35
Metformin, precocious pubarche management 46, 47, 144, 145, 147

Necdin, precocious puberty mechanisms in hypothalamic hamartoma 88

Peg3, precocious puberty mechanisms in hypothalamic hamartoma 88
Polycystic ovary syndrome (PCOS)
bone mineral density 157
dehydroepiandrosterone sulfate levels in children 46, 47
diagnosis in adolescence
criteria 139
investigations 139, 140
intrauterine growth retardation correlation 29
pathophysiology
acne 142
androgens 141
hirsutism 142
insulin resistance 142
menstrual irregularity 142, 143
presentation in adolescence 138, 139
prevalence in adolescence 149, 150
treatment in precocious pubarche
cyproterone acetate 145, 146
finasteride 146
flutamide 146
lifestyle modification 143, 144
metformin 46, 47, 144, 145, 147
spironolactone 146
weight loss 143, 144, 146
Precocious puberty
central precocious puberty
course 99, 100
definition 96
etiology 96–99
evaluation
hormonal findings 100, 101
imaging 101, 102
physical examination 100
incidence 96

congenital adrenal hyperplasia 57, 58
definition 9, 11, 126
gonadotropin secretion 9–11
hypothalamic hamartoma, *see* Hypothalamic hamartoma
long-term follow-up of women at age 43 years
body mass index 128
clinical implications 134, 135
delayed-puberty women comparison 133
dieting behavior and body dissatisfaction 130
height 127–129
physical fitness 129
psychosocial development 130–132
quality of life 132, 133
study population 127, 128
sex differences 11, 12
treatment of central precocious puberty
cyproterone acetate 104
goals 103
gonadotropin-releasing hormone agonists
auxological effects 106
body mass index outcomes 114
bone mineral density outcomes 114
clinical, hormonal, and psychological effects 105, 106
final-height effects 111–114
leuprorelin 104, 105
monitoring 108–110
overview 104
pituitary and gonadal function long-term effects 110, 111
prospects 115
psychosocial outcomes 115
randomized trials 105
side effects 106–108
triptorelin 104, 105
indications 102, 103
medroxyprogesterone acetate 104
psychosocial and behavioral aspects 102, 127
somatic and hormonal aspects 102, 103
Prostaglandin E_2, precocious puberty mechanisms in hypothalamic hamartoma 87
Puberty timing, *see also* Delayed puberty; Precocious puberty
anorexia nervosa 7
congenital adrenal hyperplasia 55, 56
endocrine disrupters in environment 8, 9
genetics 3–6
immigration effects 8
nutrition effects, *see also* Intrauterine growth retardation
critical-weight hypothesis 6, 7
fetal and perinatal nutrition 7, 8, 15
race differences 95
socioeconomic effects 2
trends over time
Netherlands 2, 3, 95, 96
United States 3

Radiation therapy, *see* Fertility preservation, female cancer patients

Sonic hedgehog (SHH), precocious puberty mechanisms in hypothalamic hamartoma 87, 88
Spironolactone, polycystic ovary syndrome management in adolescence 146
Stem cell transplantation, *see* Fertility preservation, female cancer patients

Testosterone, *see* Androgens
Transforming growth factor-α (TGF-α), precocious puberty mechanisms in hypothalamic hamartoma 85–87
Triptorelin, central precocious puberty management 104, 105
Turner's syndrome
bone mineral density effects 159
management 160

UBE3A, precocious puberty mechanisms in hypothalamic hamartoma 88